Fiona Marshall is a freelance journalist and author with a particular interest in epilepsy. She writes regularly for the UK health and medical press and has written four books, *The Natural Way: Epilepsy, Coping Successfully with Your Second Child, Coping with Postnatal Depression* and *Losing a Parent*.

YOUR CHILD SERIES

A series of books containing easy-to-follow, practical advice for the parents of children with a variety of illnesses or conditions.

Each book provides a clear overview of the situation, explaining essential information about the illness or condition and outlining the practical steps parents can take to help understand, support and care for their child, the rest of the family as well as themselves. Guiding parents through the conventional, the complementary and the alternative approaches which are available, these books cater for children of all ages, ranging from babies to teenagers, and enable the whole family to move forward in a positive way.

Titles in the Your Child series:

Your Child: Asthma by Erika Harvey
Your Child: Bullying by Jenny Alexander
Your Child: Diabetes by Catherine Steven
Your Child: Dyslexia by Robin Temple
Your Child: Eczema by Maggie Jones
Your Child: Epilepsy by Fiona Marshall

YOUR CHILD

Epilepsy
Practical and Easy-to-Follow Advice

Fiona Marshall

ELEMENT

Shaftesbury, Dorset • Boston, Massachusetts
Melbourne, Victoria

© Element Books Limited 1998
Text © Fiona Marshall 1998

First published in the UK in 1998 by
Element Books Limited
Shaftesbury, Dorset SP7 8BP

Published in the USA in 1998 by
Element Books, Inc.
160 North Washington Street
Boston, MA 02114

Published in Australia in 1998 by
Element Books and distributed
by Penguin Australia Limited
487 Maroondah Highway, Ringwood,
Victoria 3134

Cover design by Slatter-Anderson
Design by Roger Lightfoot
Typeset by Intype London Ltd
Printed and bound in Great Britain by
Creative Print and Design Wales, Ebbw Vale

British Library Cataloguing in Publication
data available

Library of Congress Cataloging in Publication
data available

ISBN 1 86204 315 9

To all families affected by epilepsy

Contents

Acknowledgements

I would like to acknowledge, with thanks, the help of the following: the British Epilepsy Association and the National Society for Epilepsy, especially Alison Iliff, Information and Education Officer for the NSE, for her help in checking the manuscript, and Jo Lawrence-King; Dr Stuart Korth, director of osteopathy of the Osteopathic Hospital for Children, London; *What Doctors Don't Tell You*, a publication by the Wallace Press; staff at the Epilepsy Liaison Service, Neuropsychiatry and Seizure Clinic, Queen Elizabeth Psychiatric Hospital, Birmingham; Caroline Thomas; researcher and author; Dr Marilyn Glenville, of the Hale Clinic, London; David Collins, SHEN therapist; Joanne Whatnall and her dynamic Epilepsy Friends Group (UK–Leicester); and Michael Barrett. I also referred to two great books on epilepsy in childhood by, respectively, Dr Richard Appleton and John M. Freeman (*see* 'Further Reading'). Above all, thanks to all the parents who so generously shared their experiences of caring for a child with epilepsy.

Introduction

Epilepsy affects an estimated 50 million people worldwide, and is mostly diagnosed in childhood – about 75 per cent of people experience their first seizure before the age of 20. It is the most common serious neurological problem affecting children.

Yet many families face difficulties in obtaining even basic facts about epilepsy, and parents are often left with many unanswered questions. How can they find out more about their child's epilepsy? Will scientific research ever find a cause for their child's type of epilepsy? Are there alternatives to drugs, such as complementary remedies? What about diet and allergies? In an era when people are taking increasing responsibility for their own health, such questions are compelling for those affected by epilepsy.

For up to 80 per cent of children, seizures are controlled by drugs, so that the majority of children with uncomplicated epilepsy have an active childhood just like anyone else's. This still means, however, that the more general problems of parenting are compounded by having a child with a long-term medical condition. And if your child's condition is more complicated, or if he or she is one of the 20–25 per cent whose epilepsy is not controlled by drugs, there may be little comfort in these statistics. The side-effects of drugs, the general quality of life, the stress of having an unwell child, anxiety about the future, what to tell friends and others – these are just some of the concerns parents face. Grief, stress, anger and guilt are all common.

Epilepsy in childhood strikes at the most important and vulnerable years of one's life when the basics of self-esteem, social relationships and learning skills are being developed. A 35-year study in Finland of how childhood epilepsy affects social and educational prospects found that people with epilepsy were less likely to go on to secondary education, had a lower socio-economic status, were less likely to be in full-time employment, and were less likely to be married or living with someone. All in all, people with epilepsy were four times more likely to feel they had poor or no control over their lives.

On the positive side, since this study was started in the mid-1960s, there have been great improvements both in the public's attitude to epilepsy and in its treatment. Moreover, while the battle continues to find effective drugs with fewer side-effects, the emphasis today is increasingly moving from seizure control in its narrowest medical sense to encompass more general improvements in quality of life. Increasing numbers of people are finding that complementary therapies can have an important part to play in this. Many parents have found that their children tend to have fewer seizures when they are more relaxed, and cope better with the seizures they do have. Natural remedies can also help parents deal with the stress of having a child with epilepsy. Some families have also found that various complementary therapies appear to improve their child's epilepsy, although it must be emphasized that conventional medication must always be maintained alongside any 'alternative' remedy, as suddenly stopping anti-epileptic drugs is life-threatening. A reputable complementary practitioner will accept that this is the case, but may have an important role to play in helping boost your child's general self-confidence.

Self-confidence is important in view of the finding that children with epilepsy are at greater risk of lowered self-esteem, and the fact that the social aspect of epilepsy is still sometimes complicated by public ignorance. Many children, afraid of bullying and social isolation, hide their condition from their playmates and peers, according to the British Epilepsy Association, and teachers, government officials, and health-care workers could all benefit from knowing more about epilepsy. According to the Epilepsy Foundation of America, it is often other people's attitudes and prejudices that prevent people with epilepsy from achieving their full potential. So friends, families, physicians, therapists, counsellors and support groups all have a role in encouraging children with epilepsy to live life to the full.

The World Health Organization (WHO) has gone so far as to say that those affected by epilepsy often have to live 'secret lives' because of ill-informed public attitudes. Recently, WHO launched 'Out of the Shadows – A Global Campaign Against Epilepsy', together with the International League Against Epilepsy (ILAE), which represents health professionals, and the International Bureau for Epilepsy (IBE), which acts for patients and their families. This campaign is aimed at improving health-care services, treatment and the social acceptance of epilepsy. This raising of awareness is particularly important in view of the fact that three out of four people in the world with epilepsy – around 30 million, mainly in developing countries – do not receive any treatment at all. And when one considers that epilepsy usually begins in childhood, this is a staggering number of untreated children. Even in developed countries, services are often under-funded, leading to rushed consultations, lack of information for parents and sometimes misdiagnosis.

The key point to remember is that epilepsy is treatable. Early diagnosis and effective medical care can make all the difference to your child's personal, educational and career prospects. A vital part of this process is simply talking more openly about epilepsy – especially vital in a child's early years, when attitudes are being formed, emotional habits learned and an education started.

'Cancer, leprosy and epilepsy were the three great unmentionables until as recently as 30 years ago,' says the ILAE President, Dr Edward Reynolds. 'Now, cancer is more openly discussed while leprosy is less of a taboo, and we would like epilepsy to go that way.'

Note: 'He' and 'she' have been used to describe your child in alternate chapters to avoid the more cumbersome 'he or she'.

Chapter One

What is Epilepsy?

Case Studies

'I just thought Laura was a very jerky baby,' says her mother, Sue. 'When she began to walk, she'd suddenly stop and her head would nod right down onto her chest, and then I realized that something wasn't right.'

Anna, mother of seven-year-old Jordan, recalls: 'I was going past Jordan's bedroom and I thought I heard something fall down so I went in. He was hanging half off the bed, his eyes were right back in his head and he was blue and shaking. I thought he was dying.'

'You can tell when she's going to go because she gets very upset and panicky for half an hour beforehand – she knows she's going to have a seizure,' says Penny, mother of Barbara, aged 11. 'If I can get her to relax and go to sleep during that time, it's much better. She still jerks in her sleep, but it doesn't seem as bad.'

Debbie says of her son Christopher, aged 17: 'His epilepsy is under control but he's a very angry adolescent. You wouldn't think so at first because he's charming and has a sense of humour, but beyond the few people he trusts, like his immediate family, he's not good at sustaining relationships. He'll string girls along and then his tolerance snaps, he has an outburst of temper, and the relationship's over. It's like normal adolesence but much worse. I know that deep down he's furious he has epilepsy.'

Frustrating and unpredictable, epilepsy continues to puzzle sufferers, their families and friends, the wider public, and even at times the medical profession. For a start there is no one simple explanation of what epilepsy actually is, because it can be so many things. It is usually defined as a tendency to have recurrent seizures (fits) caused by abnormal electrical activity in the brain (known especially in the USA, as a 'seizure disorder'). But this is no more than the baldest description of what happens on occasions to a person who has epilepsy. It describes a general symptom in the most general way. There are many types of epilepsy, and many degrees of severity.

Doctors still have limited knowledge of the underlying mechanisms which cause epilepsy. Seizures are usually viewed as signalling some form of underlying brain damage or disorder, or a genetic predisposition. But, what the condition means varies widely from individual to individual. One child's epilepsy may be so mild that even her parents do not notice it for years; another may have seizures only at night or in the morning; yet another may have frequent major tonic–clonic seizures, but find that they can be completely controlled by medication.

Some children may also have behavioural or developmental problems or an additional diagnosis such as autism, so that their parents are never sure how far the 'epilepsy' is to blame for their problems. A few parents will face the challenge of having a child who has several obvious seizures a day, and who also has an accompanying condition such as cerebral palsy, perhaps having to spend her life in a wheelchair. So epilepsy means very different things to different families. Each child reacts in a different way, and presents a unique case.

■ EPILEPSY IN THE PAST

The word 'epilepsy' come from the same root as the Greek *epilambanein*, which means 'to seize' or 'to attack'. The term may derive from a very old belief that all diseases were attacks or seizures by gods or demons. At a time when human bones were recommended as a treatment for epilepsy (burnt and crushed in a drink), Hippocrates (460–377 BC), who protested that epilepsy originated in the brain, was a solitary voice of science in a wilderness of superstition. The very first book on epilepsy, *On the Sacred Disease*, written around 400 BC, is an attack on the magic practices used to treat the condition, which Hippocrates said were just a cover for lack of knowledge and fraud.

Superstition and ignorance continued to dog epilepsy down the centuries, leading to a plethora of beliefs which ranged from demons and the full moon as causes, to weasel's stomach and stones found in swallows' stomachs as cures. In medieval England it was common to have gold or silver rings made to ward off epilepsy, which gained potency from the king's blessing. In the 15th century one remedy included passing urine into a shoe. And human blood and bones were still being recommended as treatments by respectable doctors at the beginning of the 18th century.

Beliefs about the status and powers of people with epilepsy were equally diverse. At times they were shunned because epilepsy was considered contagious, at others they were believed to have the power of prophecy – prophesying 'epileptics' formed part of a tradition of prediction encompassing many cultures, from the visions of St Paul on the road to Damascus to the shamans of Arctic Europe, who could comment on events going on 300 miles away.

The voice of rational science continued to battle against this, saying that epilepsy had nothing to do with magic practices, but needed to be treated with serious medical efforts such as diet and drugs. Galen, the 2nd-century AD Greek physician, divided the condition into three types, one of which he believed was caused by obstruction of the ventricles of the brain, and drew attention to the gastric 'aura' (the Greek word for breeze) before an attack, the sensation which seemed to rise from the stomach to the head. Physicians continued to put forward increasingly sophisticated explanations as more was discovered about the structure and workings of the brain. In the first half of the 19th century, early specialists in epilepsy painstakingly started to differentiate it from psychiatric conditions such as hysteria, insanity and somnambulism. Seizures were divided into different categories, and the first drug treatment, potassium bromide, was introduced. Since then, while it was still subject to superstitious hangovers, epilepsy has become generally medicalized, and over the past half-century doctors have gained a greater understanding of how the brain works, while scientists have manufactured a plethora of increasingly sophisticated drugs for treatment.

Stigma and epilepsy – the shameful past?
Sadly, there is still a stigma attached to epilepsy today – a stigma which has a long and somewhat murky past. For example, according to a 19th-century Italian military physician, Cesare Lombroso, the 'born criminal' and the person with epilepsy were virtually the same, sharing similar physical and psychological traits. On the other hand, he believed that both had the possibilities of being a genius, due to the 'cerebral irritability' which was believed to underlie both epilepsy and great intellectual power.

This kind of theory, which viewed people with epilepsy as different and potentially dangerous, influenced perceptions and treatment for many years. Until astonishingly recently, it was by no means uncommon for people with epilepsy to suffer imprisonment, hospitalization and incarceration in colonies, and many countries had laws affecting marriage, having children and immigration. For example, up to 1971, nine US states had laws prohibiting people with epilepsy, usually institutionalized, from marrying. And, before 1965, people with epilepsy were excluded from immigrating into the US. Behind these laws lay very old beliefs – that epilepsy was contagious, and that it was always inherited – which still sometimes cast their shadow today, although public opinion is changing as more becomes known about the condition.

THE CHILDREN'S DISEASE

From the earliest times epilepsy was also known specifically as 'the disease of children' (*paidon*) because it was so common. From at least the 3rd century BC, the ancient Greeks recognized that it started most usually in early life, especially at teething. It was also spoken of as a disease of adolesence and it was considered exceptional for it to start after the age of 20.

One of the most famous episodes of childhood epilepsy is the biblical story of Jesus casting the 'dumb spirit' out of a boy ('he fell on the ground, and wallowed foaming', St Mark, 9). Although epilepsy is not mentioned, this story portray's a classic picture of the epileptic attack in action – the 'epileptic cry' noted from the times of Hippocrates, the fall, the convulsions and the foaming at the mouth. This story was for centuries highly influential in the theories of epilepsy, lunacy and demonic possession. It also draws attention to the link between fasting and seizure control ('this kind goeth out by nothing but prayer and fasting') – a link which received attention from modern science in the form of the ketogenic diet in the 1920s and again recently (*see* chapter 4).

TYPES OF EPILEPSY AND SEIZURES

There are several different types of epilepsy and it can be a confusing business picking your way through them – even for doctors not experienced in epilepsy. For example, you may hear a hospital neurologist speak of your child having tonic–clonic seizures, the most common convulsive kind, only to have your family doctor refer to the same condition as 'grand mal' attacks (a term which is now outdated but still used).

For practical purposes, doctors usually define epilepsy in terms of the type of *seizures* people have. They generally use variations of the International Classification of Epileptic Seizures as defined by the International League Against Epilepsy, which divides seizures in childhood epilepsy into three main categories:

- *generalized seizures*, when seizure activity begins in both hemispheres of the brain simultaneously, making the child lose consciousness
- *partial (focal) seizures*, which affect part of the brain, and may or may not affect consciousness, depending on how far through the brain the seizure activity goes
- special *epilepsy syndromes*, which are groups of typical seizures and other symptoms which fall into certain recognizable patterns, making up specific types of epilepsy

■ GENERALIZED SEIZURES

The best-known type of generalized seizure is what many people think of epilepsy – the convulsive tonic–clonic seizure ('grand mal'), when the person falls to the ground and jerks dramatically. But generalized seizures can also be non-convulsive, and so subtle that a bystander might not even realize that they were occurring.

The six main types of generalized seizures are:

1 **Tonic–clonic seizures**. Most tonic–clonic seizures, the most common form, last only three to four minutes, but for the parent seeing a child experience one, this can seem like a lifetime.

'Tonic' means contracting, which is how this type of seizure begins – with your child's muscles going very tight and rigid so that she can no longer stand upright and falls to the ground. The muscles round the lungs also contract, forcing out the air and causing her to give an involuntary cry, scream or grunt (the 'epileptic cry'). The teeth also clench as the jaw muscles contract, which is why it is useless to put anything in your child's mouth to prevent injury – the tongue is most likely to be bitten at the beginning of the seizure as the teeth clamp together. Because breathing may be impaired, the oxygen in her blood is quickly used up, sometimes making her turn blue. She may also dribble saliva, lose some urine or perspire, while the pupils of the eyes dilate.

All this happens very quickly, and the phase may last for only one or two minutes. The seizure then passes into the clonic or convulsive phase, when the leg, arm and trunk muscles convulse rhythmically. This passes within a few minutes, and your child may then lie unconscious, breathing hard as colour and consciousness gradually return. After the seizure, it is quite common for her to be confused or exhausted, and to have a splitting headache or painful muscles. Rest or sleep may be needed until she is fully recovered.

2 **Tonic seizures**. Your child will go rigid and fall to the ground, without jerking. This seizure usually lasts for a few seconds.

3 **Clonic seizures**. The muscles contract rhythmically so that the legs and arms, or sometimes the whole body, jerks or twitches. These usually last up to two minutes, occasionally longer.

4 **Atonic seizures (or drop attacks)**. Your child may suddenly fall to the ground because of a loss of muscle tone. Both tonic and atonic seizures can cause head and facial injuries.

5 **Myoclonic seizures**. These seizures involve sudden muscle jerks – for example, the head may suddenly nod, or there may be an abrupt jerking of the arms and/or legs. Myoclonic attacks may happen on their own or with other generalized seizures such as absence seizures.

6 **Absence seizures**. Almost always seen in childhood, these may be slightly more common in girls. Previously known as 'petit mal', they are short periods when consciousness is absent, due to interruptions in normal brain activity. Your child may simply go blank for a few moments, stare, blink

rapidly, or make chewing movements. Absence seizures begin and end abruptly, and may last only a few seconds, so that people around, and even your child herself, may be unaware that she has had a seizure. Some children have hundreds or even thousands a day.

■ PARTIAL (FOCAL) SEIZURES

These begin at a localized point in the brain, and may also spread throughout the whole brain, becoming a secondarily generalized seizure. Your child may or may not lose consciousness, depending on whether the seizure is simple or complex.

Simple partial seizures (sometimes also known as Jacksonian seizures after the British neurologist John Hughlings Jackson, 1835–1911) affect a small area of the brain. Your child will remain awake without her consciousness being affected, so long as the seizure activity remains within a small area. If the seizure does spread over both halves (hemispheres) of the brain, so that she loses consciousness, the seizure is known as a *secondarily generalized seizure*. In this case, the simple partial seizure is also the *aura* or warning of a more widespread attack. Auras take different forms, depending on which part of the brain is affected (*see* 'Seizures and brain structure' below) but common ones include a feeling of nausea rising upward from the stomach, and a feeling of fear.

Complex partial seizures occur when the activity spreads to a larger area of the brain, so affecting your child's consciousness more. The way in which this happens depends on which part of the brain is touched by the seizure, as explained below.

■ SEIZURES AND BRAIN STRUCTURE

The brain is divided into two hemispheres, and generalized seizures begin simultaneously in both halves. It is further sub-divided into four lobes – temporal, frontal, parietal and occipital

– and partial seizures may start from any of these lobes. Depending on which part of the brain is affected – most commonly the temporal or frontal lobes – the child experiences different sensations.

- **The temporal lobe** controls understanding, memories, emotions, smells and tastes. If the seizure begins here, your child may experience unpleasant smells or tastes, or may feel giddy and sick. If the seizure involves the amygdala and hippocampus, areas of the brain connected with the emotions, she may experience fear. And, because this part of the brain controls memory, another common feeling is *déjà vu* (the feeling that this has all happened before).
- **The frontal lobe** controls movement, speech and emotions. If a seizure begins in this part of the brain, your child may only feel a twitching or jerking of her arms or legs, or eye movements.
- **The parietal lobe** is responsible for perception and body sensations. Seizures which begin here may start with tingling or pins and needles in some part of the body, for example down one side.
- **The occipital lobe** is responsible for sight. If seizures involve this part of the brain, your child may see bright flashing lights for a few seconds, perhaps to one side of her vision.

Status epilepticus

Status epilepticus is the term used when seizures last for at least 30 minutes, or happen one after another for a period of 30 minutes or more with no return of consciousness in between. This is a medical emergency, as there is a risk of brain damage or even death from a shortage of oxygen to the brain. Anti-epileptic drugs need to be injected into the muscles or the veins.

There are two main sorts of status epilepticus: convulsive, which involve tonic–clonic seizures, and non-convulsive, when the person has absence or staring spells, or confusion, for half an hour or more.

When does a 'normal' seizure become status epilepticus? As a general guideline, you should seek urgent medical help if your child has a second or third seizure without regaining consciousness, if a seizure lasts more than five minutes, or if your child has a longer than usual convulsive phase of a seizure (about two minutes longer than usual).

EPILEPSY SYNDROMES

The term 'epilepsy syndrome' is used when seizures follow certain recognizable patterns or a typical course. This sounds very neat, but like epilepsy in general, syndromes are a complex subject, and clear diagnosis is not always possible, especially where several complex features may be involved, such as the Lennox–Gastaut syndrome.

One reason why doctors classify syndromes like this is to have a clearer idea not just of proper treatment, but of the likely outcome, or prognosis. Most syndromes start in childhood, even between certain typical ages; and, while some have serious long-term implications, others are much less serious and may be outgrown, also at certain ages. However, many of these serious syndromes are very rare. It is more likely that your child will have a condition in which her seizures can be controlled.

Benign rolandic epilepsy of childhood (BREC)

(Also known as benign partial epilepsy with centro-temporal or rolandic spikes)
How common: A very common type of partial epilepsy, BREC comprises 15–20 per cent of all childhood epilepsy cases.
Age: 2–14, but more usually 4–10. More common in boys.
Cause: Uncertain – there may be a genetic component.
Seizures: May begin with a feeling of pins and needles at one side of the mouth and spread to one side of the face, and may involve jerking or paralysis. They may also involve one hand,

or spread down one side of the body, or become a tonic, clonic or tonic–clonic convulsion down one side of the body and face. Speech problems and salivation may happen during the seizure, but the child remains conscious.

Other effects: BREC is said to be 'benign' because it is usually outgrown by adolescence, and the child's intellect remains unaffected.

Treatment: Seizures may be infrequent, or happen more often at night or on waking, so the child may not need treatment; but if she does, BREC responds well to carbamazepine (*see* page 66).

Prognosis: Good – the child usually outgrows BREC by puberty.

Juvenile myoclonic epilepsy (JME)

(Also known as Janz syndrome)

How common: The most common epilepsy syndrome in teenagers.

Age: 8–18, more usually 12–16, often around puberty.

Cause: Believed to be genetic.

Seizures: Usually take the form of mild jerking (myoclonic jerks) of the arms or legs, often as the child is dropping off to sleep or waking up. Occasionally, these may pass on to generalized tonic–clonic seizures, and some people may also have absence seizures.

Other effects: Photosensitivity is common. Lack of sleep or (in teenagers) alcohol or periods may trigger seizures.

Treatment: Usually quite well controlled by a drug such as sodium valproate (*see* page 66).

Prognosis: Good.

West syndrome

(Also known as infantile spasms or salaam spasms.)

How common: Rare – 3 per cent of all childhood epilepsy cases.

Age: In the first year of life, often between three and six months.

Cause: Often not known, but may include: developmental brain problems; brain damage caused by birth injury, meningitis or accidents; or abnormalities of metabolism such as low blood sugar or amino acid problems.

Seizures: Take the form of spasms, most often when the child is waking up or dropping off to sleep. Your baby will draw her knees up, bending in two, perhaps with the head bent forward too (the 'salaam' gesture), and gives a short cry. Less often, she may throw her head and limbs backwards and out, or the spasms may only affect one side of the body or just consist of head or eyelid movements.

Other effects: Spasms may sometimes be mistaken for colic. The main difference is that colic does not show as a series of spasms, while infantile spasms tend to occur in bouts of anything from five to 50. In colic, your child will also have her knees drawn up beneath her, but will tend to cry persistently, being typically red-faced and screaming, and hard to soothe.

Treatment: Various, involving a range of drugs; ketogenic diet (*see* pages 79–84). Seizures tend to be hard to control.

Prognosis: Sadly, poor. Though not common, West syndrome does carry a risk of mortality, however, this would need to be discussed on an individual basis with a doctor. While this form of epilepsy usually disappears between the ages of two and four, the child's development is often retarded. Shortly after the first spasms begin, she may stop progressing and may even seem to go backward, losing skills already acquired, such as sitting and babbling. Only around 10–20 per cent of children with West syndrome will be normal mentally, and around half or more go on to develop other forms of epilepsy, especially Lennox–Gastaut syndrome.

Lennox–Gastaut syndrome

How common: Rare – 1 per cent of all childhood epilepsy cases.
Age: From around two to six, but may start up to eight.
Cause: This syndrome is often seen in children with developmental brain problems or brain damage, for example after

meningitis, but a definite cause is only found in about half of all children.

Seizures: May be of several kinds – atonic (falling down), tonic and atypical absence. Many children have to wear protective headgear to prevent injury.

Other effects: This is the most common difficult-to-treat epilepsy, frustrating for medical practitioners and parents alike, and it can be devastating for parents to accept and manage.

Treatment: May involve a combination of drugs as seizures can be very hard to control. Newer medications and the ketogenic diet (*see* pages 79–84) may help. Surgery (corpus callosotomy, *see* page 73) is sometimes used.

Prognosis: Poor. Seizures may lessen in frequency but the child usually suffers from developmental delay and learning difficulties.

Landau–Kleffner syndrome (LKS)

How common: Rare.

Age: Often starts from ages two to seven.

Cause: Not known.

Seizures: Affect around 75 per cent of children with LKS, and may often be mild and easily treated. Most children have eye-blinking and head-dropping, and occasionally generalized tonic–clonic seizures.

Other effects: Usually, children are normal intellectually before LKS starts. The syndrome affects their speech – when children do not respond, parents may blame lack of attention, day-dreaming or deafness. In time, your child may even lose her ability to recognize environmental sounds such as a dog barking or the doorbell ringing. There may also be developmental problems and psychomotor and behavioural difficulties. Many children are misdiagnosed as having hearing problems, and the condition may also be confused with autism. Among sufferers, boys outnumber girls by two to one.

Treatment: Corticosteroids (*see* page 64); a range of antiepileptics; surgery (*see* pages 70–74).

Prognosis: Good for seizure control (seizures may disappear by 15–16), but poorer for language recovery.

Sturge–Weber syndrome (SWS)

How common: Rare.
Age: Birth or later in the first year.
Cause: The blood vessels in the brain fail to develop properly in the baby early in pregnancy, although it is not known why. Babies have a dark red birthmark, usually on the forehead, which may extend over the eye and face.
Seizures: These occur in 60–90 per cent of all children with SWS, and are usually partial motor seizures involving jerks of one side of the body. The seizures may become generalized or involve other types such as drop attacks, myoclonic or infantile spasms.
Other effects: The abnormal blood vessels cause shrinkage (atrophy) of the underlying brain, causing seizures, and weakness and paralysis of the opposite side of the body. They may also involve the eye area, causing hemiaropia (inability to see out of the weaker eye) or glaucoma (increased pressure in the eye due to an abnormality in the draining of the eye fluid). Children may be normal intellectually, or have mental retardation and learning difficulties.
Treatment: Drugs, often in combination. Surgery of the affected part of the brain can help in some cases (*see* pages 70–74). Glaucoma can be treated if it develops, and laser treatment may be very effective for the birthmarks.
Prognosis: Unfortunately, this kind of epilepsy can be hard to control with medication. Generally, the worse the epilepsy, the more severe the child's difficulties.

Rasmussen's syndrome

How common: Very rare.
Age: 1–14.

Cause: May be partly inherited. It may be a result of problems with the immune system involving an auto-immune process in which the body produces antibodies which destroy its own brain cells.

Seizures: Generalized tonic–clonic or focal seizures or a condition called epilepsia partalis continua (continuous focal epilepsy), in which a part of the body such as hand, face or foot may continuously jerk.

Other effects: Rasmussen's syndrome has variable effects, but can be very destructive mentally, leaving a child intellectually damaged.

Treatment: Surgery, removal of half of the brain (hemispherectomy) which stops seizures and allows more normal mental development (*see* page 73).

Prognosis: While surgery may have side-effects, prognosis may be even poorer without it.

▓ OTHER CONDITIONS WHICH CAN BE MISTAKEN FOR EPILEPSY

Epilepsy is dogged by misdiagnosis – paediatric neurologist John Stephenson, of Glasgow, estimates that about half of his referrals have been misdiagnosed as having epilepsy. There is a wide range of other conditions which may cause attacks similar to epileptic seizures, the most common of which are described below.

▓ Reflex anoxic seizures (pallid syncopal attacks)

These usually affect children aged one to four but can occur in older children. It is a faint triggered by a bad fright or by pain, which causes the vagus nerve to slow down the heart. As a result your child may go limp and pale and may have a brief clonic (jerking) convulsion. She quickly recovers, perhaps with some crying or sleepiness. These attacks do no damage to the brain or heart, and do not need treatment, beyond keeping your child's head down at the time of the faint.

Breath-holding attacks

These tend to occur mostly in children aged one to three, quite often as a result of a tantrum or being told off. The angry child holds her breath, and, after a few seconds, turns blue from lack of oxygen and passes out. Because of the reduced oxygen supply she may jerk slightly and perhaps wet herself. However, passing out solves the problem as she automatically starts breathing again and is back to normal within a few minutes. Children usually outgrow breath-holding attacks by four or five.

Fainting (syncope or vasovagal attacks)

Faints may happen if your child has been standing for a long time, is too warm, is unwell with a stomach upset or infection, or has had a bad shock or sudden pain – trapping fingers in a door is a typical example. They tend to be more common in teenage girls. The brain is short of blood and your child feels dizzy and sick, may go very pale, and falls to the ground.

The confusion with seizures may arise because your child may jerk briefly as a result of the blood shortage to the brain (which is why it is best to keep the head lowered in a faint). Moreover, the symptoms of some partial seizures may resemble those of a faint. However, a fainting child usually goes limp after initial jerking (as opposed to having convulsions or going rigid) and tends to recover more quickly than after a seizure.

Migraine

Migraine resembles epilepsy in that brainwave patterns may show abnormalities during the attack. Like some seizures, it is sometimes preceded by an aura, although in migraine the aura tends to last for longer.

Hyperventilation

Hyperventilation, or breathing too deeply or quickly, may happen if your child is feeling nervous or panicky. Too much carbon dioxide is breathed out, reducing the acidity of the blood, which in turn influences the nerves in muscle groups, and may cause spasms, tingling and blackouts.

Non-epileptic attacks (NEAs; pseudoseizures or psychological seizures)

These seizures tend to take place for psychological rather than clinical reasons, and eclectroencephalograms (EEGs) will probably be normal, although your child may not always be aware that the attacks are psychological. NEAs are more common in girls than in boys, and in teenagers than younger children. Psychological counselling may be needed, not medication. However, a child can have both epileptic and non-epileptic attacks.

Febrile convulsions

Some babies and young children have what look like seizures when they run a high temperature, for example when suffering a bad ear infection. Unless there is an underlying predisposition to epilepsy, it is believed that febrile convulsions are not a form of epilepsy. Terrifying as these often are, they cause no brain damage, and the child almost always recovers fully and usually outgrows them by age four or five. A tendency to febrile convulsions tends to be inherited, and affects 2–4 per cent of children, more commonly girls.

Daydreaming and absence seizures

Absence seizures, when the child blanks out for a few seconds or longer, are the type which are typically mistaken for daydreaming. The differences are outlined below.

Absence seizure	Daydreaming
Your child cannot be roused.	Your child is easily roused, eg by a touch on arm.
Social activities are interrupted.	Your child is less likely to daydream when occupied (eg eating, talking, playing).
May occur several times a day, at any time.	May only occur in specific situations, eg at school.
Tend to start abruptly.	Your child drifts into dreaming more gradually.
May not last beyond 15 seconds.	May go on until your child is distracted.
Your child does not remember conversation.	Your child is vaguely aware of conversations which have been going on around her.

■ CAUSES OF EPILEPSY

Why has my child got epilepsy? Did I do something wrong in my pregnancy? Was it the time she fell off her tricycle and I didn't take her to hospital? A diagnosis of epilepsy in a child often produces much heart-searching and guilt among parents, who may search exhaustively for causes, delving into their own past behaviour for a possible reason. This process forms an important part of coming to terms with, or grieving over, your child's epilepsy. However, in up to 75 per cent of cases no cause can be found, and it is in any case highly unlikely that the condition arises out of anything you have done.

This type of epilepsy, when no cause can be found, is known as *idiopathic epilepsy* idiopathic simply means 'of unknown cause'. *Cryptogenic epilepsy* is the term used when a cause is suspected but none can be found, and when a cause is known – such as underlying abnormality in the brain structure, infection (eg meningitis) or head injury – it is *symptomatic epilepsy*. However, these divisions are changing somewhat under the impact of

modern investigative methods such as scans. A child who 20
years ago might have been diagnosed with idiopathic epilepsy
may now be found to have a tiny developmental abnormality of
the brain, which would have been missed by previous conventional techniques. New light may also be thrown on idiopathic
epilepsy by genetic factors.

Known causes of epilepsy tend to be fairly rare. For example,
sometimes it follows a difficulty during pregnancy or birth,
although thanks to modern obstetrics babies are very carefully
monitored for lack of oxygen (anoxia) during delivery, making
this a far less common cause than before. Other risk factors
which may affect the baby include the mother having viral or
bacterial infections during pregnancy, excess alcohol consump-
tion and illegal drug use. These have occasionally been
associated with a child who has epilepsy, although parents certainly should not agonize over whether an extra drink or so on
the odd occasion caused their child's epilepsy. Unborn babies
are mostly very resilient, and in most cases no cause for the
epilepsy can be found.

Other factors are toxins, such as lead poisoning or aluminium
toxicity, or chemical injury to the brain. Seizures may also be
triggered by blood chemical abnormalities such as low calcium,
magnesium or glucose if a child has a low seizure threshold.

Finally, although most children are quite resilient, a head
injury may occasionally result in seizures, especially if it is severe
or followed by a long period of unconsciousness. Brain tumours
are a rare cause of epilepsy in children – around one in 100.

Causes may vary according to how old your child is at the
time she develops epilepsy. Generally speaking, seizures in babies
and toddlers are thought most often to be a result of brain injury
around the time of birth, congenital central nervous system
malformations or abnormalities in the metabolism. In later childhood, they are more likely to be caused by severe infection of
the central nervous system such as meningitis or encephalitis
(inflammation of the brain), genetic epilepsies or neurodegener-

ative disorders. In contrast, the most common causes of seizures in adults include brain injury and stroke.

The vaccine debate

Vaccines have been blamed for causing neurological damage and epilepsy, but this is a controversial issue. Vaccines implicated include those for diphtheria, tetanus, pertussis or whooping cough (DTP), and for measles, mumps and rubella (MMR).

According to British consultant paediatric neurologist and author Dr Richard Appleton, nearly all the medical evidence suggests that whooping cough vaccine does *not* cause epilepsy. 'In fact, there is a much greater risk of brain damage and epilepsy occurring in a young child (one less than two or three years old) who has NOT been vaccinated against whooping cough (also called pertussis) than of a child of a similar age suffering brain damage because of the vaccine,' he says in his book *Your Child's Epilepsy* (*see* 'Further Reading'). 'Vaccination has been so effective in controlling childhood illnesses that we have almost forgotten how dangerous some of these infections can be.' A very few children have appeared to develop epilepsy within 24 hours of having a vaccination, but this may be from extremely rare freak conditions such as a particular batch of vaccines being contaminated, and is no reason to avoid vaccination, he says. A number of large-scale medical research studies have failed to find any definitive link between the pertussis vaccine and brain damage, and figures show that the risk of brain damage and death is far greater from whooping cough than from vaccines.

On the other side of the debate, the UK alternative health publication *What Doctors Don't Tell You* (*WDDTY*) claims that parents have good reason for anxiety about immunizations. *WDDTY* published a report on a huge study of 500,000 children by the US Centers for Disease Control and Prevention in Atlanta, which apparently showed that the seizure rate was three times the norm for children receiving the DTP and MMR jabs. This evidence was not made public because of government programmes promoting vaccines, according to *WDDTY*. And, according to Dr Harris Coulter, medical historian and critic of conventional medicine, epilepsy increased dramatically around 1945, when the USA started its mass vaccination programme. It is recognized that vaccination causes a slight degree of encephalitis in 1 in 100,000 cases, but Coulter believes it may happen about once in five cases. The child may recover completely, but may also suffer long-term damage which can take the form of epilepsy.

For more details on whether your child should have routine immunizations, see pages 111–12.

The genetic question

Increasingly, research is focusing on genetic explanations for epilepsy, and many doctors believe these may play more of a part than was previously thought. Certain types of epilepsy are known to have a higher genetic risk than others JME (*see* page 11). It is also known that epilepsy can be caused by some genetic conditions such as tuberous sclerosis, a rare congenital disease with abnormal cell development which affects the brain, other organs and the central nervous system.

But while epilepsy seems to run in some families, a genetic predisposition does not necessarily mean that a child will develop seizures. It may be that there needs to be an additional triggering factor, such as another gene, a severe illness such as encephalitis or a bad head injury. Much still remains to be discovered about how the genes interrelate to produce the condition – a highly complex area. For example, researchers are looking at how genetics may contribute to problems with brain development before birth, such as what are known as neuronal migration disorders, when brain cells fail to develop in the right place early in pregnancy. Some children with epilepsy are born with dysplasias, pockets of neurones that are in the wrong places, and scientists are investigating how genes may operate during the unborn baby's development to influence the placing and connecting of these neurones.

Epilepsy and genetic research

In a study of the families of nearly 2,000 people with epilepsy, a genetic link has been found for partial epilepsy, in which seizures begin in a specific part of the brain. Professor Ruth Ottman, who headed the research at the Comprehensive Epilepsy Center of the Columbia-Presbyterian Medical Center, and her colleagues found a specific gene which may be responsible for some cases of partial epilepsy, though other factors such as environmental or other genetic influences may often be required in order for the gene to cause epilepsy.

Researchers at the University College London Medical School have evidence that another specific gene, 15, appears to cause susceptibility to JME in 65 per cent of the families studied. The research could lead to drugs being targeted at particular receptors, so leading to more effective seizure control and reduced side-effects of medication, says Dr Frances Elmslie, Training Fellow for Action Research, which funded the project.

Epilepsy and brain development research

A study by the Washington University School of Medicine, St Louis, has suggested that some epilepsy might be triggered by problems in the unborn baby's brain with neurotrophin-4 (NT-4), a protein normally thought to control cells in the part of the cerebral cortex which controls thought and speech. Research showed that problems with NT-4 seemed to result in abnormalities similar to those seen in epilepsy and some forms of mental retardation. This kind of highly specialized research shows the kind of detail that may need to be investigated before the causes of epilepsy can be better understood.

■ LINKS WITH OTHER CONDITIONS

Children are more likely to have epilepsy if they have certain other conditions affecting the brain, such as cerebral palsy, autism and learning difficulties. But this does not mean that epilepsy causes these conditions, or vice versa – in such cases, an underlying brain dysfunction or damage has caused both epilepsy and the other condition. A child with an additional condition or conditions may unfortunately have a more severe form of epilepsy, which is more difficult to control (sometimes known as 'epilepsy plus').

Some research has shown that people with epilepsy are more likely to suffer from depression. However, this can be interpreted in different ways. In the past, especially, depression may have been a response to less sophisticated medications. Depression may still be a side-effect of some drugs, or of nutrient deficiencies caused by drugs or other factors. Some children also experience depression as part of the build-up to a seizure (a process known medically as prodrome). Or they may be depressed at having epilepsy and the limitations and stigma they feel it brings – even if these are more perceived than real.

Autism and Asberger's syndrome

Autism and Asberger's syndrome are still being defined and differentiated, but they are believed to be neurological disorders centring round difficulties relating to and communicating with others.

About 30 per cent of children with autism also have epilepsy. One type of epilepsy which is sometimes confused with autism is LKS (*see* page 13). LKS and autism, while not related, seem similar in that children may often start to speak in single words or two-word sentences but then stop around the age of 18 months. To confuse the issue even more, children with autism often have abnormal EEGs, as do children with epilepsy, and it may take detailed tests to tell whether the activity recorded is epileptic or not.

Cerebral palsy

Cerebral palsy involves damage to a person's motor control, and about one in three children with cerebral palsy will also have epilepsy.

Learning difficulties

Up to 50 per cent of children with severe learning difficulties also have epilepsy, and this is discussed more fully in chapter 5.

WHY DO SEIZURES HAPPEN?

It is the nature of epilepsy that children are 'seized' by attacks which seem to come out of the blue. But are seizures that random? What factors actually set the abnormal brain activity in motion?

The brain is a delicate complex of activity which works on electricity. Its nerve cells or neurones maintain a constant, regulated flow of communication by 'firing' tiny electrical impulses along connecting fibres called axons. Seizures happen when this normal interaction between brain cells is disrupted by unusually intense electrical activity. The level of excitation varies depending on the individual's seizure threshold, the level at which the brain will have a seizure.

If this seizure threshold is attacked too strongly by certain stimuli – such as high fever or a bout of drinking – a seizure may be the result. In fact, given too much stimulus, anyone can have a seizure even if they do not have epilepsy – a classic example is a seizure after heavy drinking, which is due to alcohol withdrawal.

Children with epilepsy have a lower than normal seizure threshold, making the brain cells more likely to 'fire' at a lower level of stimulus. Various factors affect one's seizure threshold, including age – the younger the person, the lower the threshold may be, making a seizure more likely, which may help explain why children often outgrow epilepsy as their brain matures. Other factors affecting the threshold are fairly fixed underlying influences such as genetic inheritance and brain scarring, and more temporary ones such as lack of sleep, excitement or fever. Some of these factors may interact to lower the threshold and produce seizures – for example, fever combined with an underlying brain scar.

■ SEIZURE TRIGGERS

Some children are more likely to have seizures in certain situations. A few may even manipulate this to their own advantage by inducing (or threatening) a seizure when faced with something they do not want to do! But childhood is also the ideal time to learn ways of managing situations in which a seizure is more likely, as opposed to avoiding them.

One seizure trigger, of course, is simply not taking one's antiepileptic medication. This can happen accidentally, if you or your child forgets, or deliberately, if she rebels. Illness will also affect how well a drug is absorbed – an obvious example is an attack of vomiting and diarrhoea. A child who has a bad cold or is feeling generally unwell may also be more likely to have a seizure as her overall resistance is lowered.

Other seizure triggers include:

- **Stress, excitement and emotional upset**. These may lower your child's resistance to seizures by affecting her sleep or eating habits, or perhaps by causing her to hyperventilate. Like adults, children may experience stress from relationships, in the family or at school, and there is information on how to manage this stress in chapter 2.
- **Boredom**. Research has demonstrated that someone who is enjoyably occupied is less likely to have a seizure – an interesting example of the mind and body link, which is explored more in chapter 4.
- **Tiredness**. Lack of sleep is known to change the brain's patterns of electrical activity and can trigger seizures. Regular sleeping patterns are important in maintaining health generally, although they may be more difficult to achieve with babies and toddlers and again with teenagers. More advice on

encouraging good sleep patterns in your child is given in chapter 5.

- **Raised temperature**. A high temperature may make some children more likely to have seizures, although this is not to be confused with febrile convulsions, when children have non-epileptic convulsions owing to a high temperature (*see* chapter 5).

- **Alcohol**. Too much alcohol can trigger seizures, and some anti-epileptic medication may also make a person more sensitive to its effects. Chapters 2 and 5 provide guidance on how to encourage moderation in your teenager.

- **Dietary factors**. Like sleep, regular meals are an important part of overall health, particularly in growing children. This may have added significance in children with epilepsy in that many seizures take place at a time when blood sugar is low.

    Some stimulants may trigger seizures by suddenly changing the body's metabolism. These include tea, coffee, chocolate, sugar, sweets, soft drinks, excess salt, spices and animal protein.

    Some parents have found that an allergic reaction to certain foods such as white flour seems to trigger off seizures in their children. Certain nutrient shortages have also been linked with seizures, such as lack of calcium. For more on good nutrition, see chapters 2 and 4.

- **Periods**. Some teenage girls find that their seizures increase around the time of their period. This is called catamenial epilepsy and may be caused by changes in levels of the hormones oestrogen and progesterone, perhaps in combination with increased fluid retention and changes in the levels of anti-epileptic drugs in the blood.

- **Heat**. Very warm weather, especially if it comes on suddenly, overheated rooms and hot baths or showers may be seizure triggers for a few children.

- **Medicine**. Some children have had seizures triggered for example by cough medicine, but this may be a highly individual reaction.

Television, videos and flashing lights

There has been quite a lot of publicity about the possibility of television and videos triggering seizures. In one of the worst recent incidents, hundreds of children were reported as suffering nausea and seizures when a Japanese television programme showed a monster flashing strobe lighting from its eyes. In the USA, some people with epilepsy are campaigning to get television networks to ban the use of flashing lights in commercials and other programmes – the so-called 'strobe effect', which involves fast scene changes emphasized by the use of a white screen. Some people's seizures can also be triggered by rapidly changing colours and fast-moving shadows on television. In the UK in 1993, the Independent Television Commission brought in regulations preventing frequent flickering and flashing images on television programmes and advertisements following complaints that a commercial had triggered epileptic seizures.

Flashing lights are so well known as a seizure trigger that it almost approaches the status of an epilepsy myth, but this type of *photosensitive epilepsy* is in fact quite rare, affecting only about 4 per cent of children with epilepsy. It is more common among girls.

Photosensitive epilepsy is one of the reflex epilepsies – conditions in which a child's seizure is a reflex action to a certain stimulus, similar to the way the lower leg jerks when your knee is hit in a certain spot. Reflex epilepsy is not just about flashing lights, however. A few children may have seizures triggered by other stimuli, including certain sounds such as traffic, or certain patterns such as squares, lines or even printed words.

Many children spend quite a lot of time watching television and videos, so any seizures could be coincidental. It may be worth restricting their vewing, however. Other ways of minimizing photosensitivity when watching television include:

• watching in a well-lit room
• sitting at least 2.5 metres away and at an angle from the television
• using a high-frequency (100Mhz) television

- making sure the set is working properly, as faulty screens can cause problems
- some photosensitive reactions can be minimized by covering one eye
- using special sunglasses, which are available via epilepsy support organizations

Flashing lights should not be a problem unless they flash at a frequency of 15–60 flashes a second (ordinary lights in clubs often flash much slower than this). You can check in advance which nightclubs and disc jockeys use dangerous levels of lighting.

SUDDEN UNEXPECTED DEATH IN EPILEPSY (SUDEP)

The risk of premature death in people with epilepsy is about two to four times greater than in the population in general, and is greatest among children, young adults and in the first ten years after diagnosis. When this happens without warning, it is known as sudden unexpected death in epilepsy (SUDEP), and there are currently believed to be between 200 and 500 cases in the UK alone every year. Many health professionals do not tell their patients about SUDEP, but there has been growing feeling among some specialists and people affected by epilepsy that parents have the right to be informed about the risks it poses, just as they are with asthma. However, so little is known about SUDEP that it is not even possible to give advice on how to avoid it.

What research has been done (largely on adults) shows that it is more prevalent with uncontrolled epilepsy and tonic–clonic seizures, and among young men. It seems likely that there are varying causes, or a combination of causes, and these are currently believed to be connected with changes in heart rhythms due to electrical changes in the brain during a seizure, and possibly with the release of certain hormones as well as the stopping of breathing during a seizure.

So what can parents do?

- Press for effective and prompt medical treatment for your child's epilepsy.
- Get seizures under control as much as possible.
- Avoid sudden drug withdrawal.
- Ensure that your child takes her medication regularly.
- If you are particularly concerned, attend a first-aid course where mouth-to-mouth resuscitation is covered.

However, it is worth remembering that SUDEP is extremely rare, and tends to affect people slightly later in life (most commonly between the ages of 20 and 30), so that being informed about SUDEP need not mean taking on a huge burden of worry. It will probably not affect your child.

■ THE PROGNOSIS – DO CHILDREN OUTGROW EPILEPSY?

Unfortunately, there is no way to predict whether a particular child's seizures will disappear in later life. But, on the positive side, it is important to realize that around 30–40 per cent of all children who develop epilepsy before they are 16 *will* outgrow their epilepsy before adulthood.

Outgrowing epilepsy is more common in some forms than others. For example, 70–75 per cent of children will stop having absence seizures by the age of 14–16. BREC also tends to be outgrown in the teenage years. Sadly, other forms of epilepsy have a much poorer outlook, for example West syndrome and Lennox–Gastaut syndrome, which account for around 20 per cent of all epilepsy.

One major school of medical thought has traditionally emphasized starting drug treatment sooner rather than later in the belief that early treatment makes for a better prognosis and may help stop epilepsy in later life. Some doctors have also wondered if anti-epileptic drugs may somehow help 'cure' the condition in the long-term, as well as suppressing seizures in the short term, but this remains no more than an interesting speculation for the time being. Some doctors also now believe that much precious time can be wasted waiting for a child to outgrow epilepsy and that surgery should•be considered earlier rather than later, as a successful outcome will make the most of a child's formative years.

On the other hand, some research suggests that in some children recently diagnosed epilepsy may sometimes remit (seem to stop spontaneously) even without being treated (*see* pages 63–4). Of course, this should not be seen as encouragement to throw out all your child's medications and hope for the best, but many children can be successfully weaned off drugs so long as it is done under the supervision of a physician. There is more on this in chapter 3.

Chapter Two

Helping Your Child

Overprotection is the biggest single issue in epilepsy, according to the eminent British epileptologist Dr Stephen Brown. Sometimes known as the 'benevolent overreaction' in medical circles, overprotection, which is surprisingly common even in well-controlled epilepsy, is notoriously counterproductive. The consequences can be serious, and lasting, affecting a child into adulthood: dependency, hypochondria, low self-esteem, underachievement and immaturity have all been catalogued.

It is a daunting list – and one which might make parents feel somewhat helpless and angry. After all, faced with a diagnosis of epilepsy, it may sometimes seem as if there is nothing you can do except go all out to protect your child as best you can from this bewildering affliction. Witnessing a seizure, living with the unpredictability and worrying about how epilepsy may limit your child's life are all likely to make you feel frustrated and powerless. But in fact, there is plenty that you can do to help your child learn to deal with his epilepsy on his own terms, and develop emotional, intellectual and practical independence. This includes being realistic about your child and his potential, as well as encouraging him to fulfil himself. Learning to recognize individual limitations forms an important part of developing maturity, health and wellbeing for everyone.

These days, all parents tend to worry more, and to be more protective. Due to the increase in traffic, and the less common but well-publicized 'stranger danger', children generally are more restricted. Obviously, these fears have more resonances for parents of children with epilepsy, but it remains true that these fears have to be seen in context, as part of an age when all children have less freedom, and need to be taught certain skills to cope accordingly.

Research shows that it is not the epilepsy itself which has the impact, but the attitudes of other people around it. It is in these early years that attitudes are formed which can last a lifetime. Parents can help by ensuring that their own attitudes are as positive as possible – not just their attitudes to epilepsy, but to life in general. You can also help your child by helping yourself, and by looking after your own life, health and wellbeing.

■ HOW DOES A DIAGNOSIS OF EPILEPSY AFFECT A FAMILY?

Case Study
The whole family was shocked when Natalie's epilepsy was confirmed by the hospital neurologist, and her relationship with her father suffered in particular – he was depressed, irritable and unable to cope with the diagnosis. He went through a phase of ignoring Natalie, and took out his negative feelings on his wife Jocelyn.

It may take time for the whole family to come to terms with a diagnosis of epilepsy, and it is quite common for normal relationship patterns to be upset for a while. A diagnosis has been described as a bereavement and certain similar stages of mourning have been documented – shock, denial, anger, depression and a period of grief before final acceptance. However, reactions may vary widely. Some people may be relieved to find out what the problem is, and to start treatment. A medical label can sometimes be a help in that it gives you something definite to deal with.

Many families tend to be governed by a series of unstated

'laws', with certain standards being assumed as the norm – sports prowess, high academic achivement or perfect health – and a diagnosis of epilepsy easily upsets the family dynamics. Ted, for example, felt (wrongly as it turned out) that Sam's epilepsy would stop him playing football and so was something of a disgrace and 'unmanly'. Another set of parents had high academic expectations for their daughter, which they feared epilepsy would blight.

It is true that in some cases families have to adjust to changed perceptions of the child. 'You go through a period of grieving, because you've not got the child you thought you had,' as one mother put it.

You may find that your relationship as partners and parents goes through an upheaval, with more frequent quarrels, or a loss of interest in sex. Some people even keep their child's condition a secret from their partners – one family were out on a walk when their youngest child had a seizure; this was the first time her father had ever seen her have one, or realized that she had epilepsy. Obviously, this is an extreme case, but it does demonstrate how easy it can sometimes be not to talk about vital issues even to your nearest and dearest.

Talking to other people can also be very healing. Epilepsy support organizations can put you in touch with other parents in the same situation, although some people initially feel too raw for this and need more time to come to terms with events in private. Others may want more structured counselling with someone impartial, who can help them express their feelings of loss and confusion, and their own needs, in a supportive environment; again, an epilepsy organization, your family doctor or a national counselling association may be able to help.

Brothers and sisters

As with any long-term condition, it can be hard not to treat the 'sick' child differently, particularly when it comes to discipline. Occasionally parents overcompensate, or spoil the child, as a way of dealing with their anger or disappointment or through fear of triggering a seizure if they thwart him too much. But this is a false dynamic, which may end up creating more insecurity both for the child with epilepsy and for his siblings, who will naturally feel excluded, jealous and resentful. Within reason, it is better to give the same attention and discipline to all the children, and to realize that it is a normal part of loving parenting to feel angry, frustrated or even tearful at times.

Your other children may also not understand epilepsy – they may be frightened of it or afraid that they will catch it – so it is very important to include them in any explanations you give about the condition. They may equally be very loving and protective, and want to take an active share in helping with their brother or sister in the event of a seizure – for example, making sure the area around him is clear and removing dangerous objects, getting help from an adult and reassuring him. It is an area which can bring its own rewards – and pains.

Case Study
'It's quite hard – most families ask the older child to look after the younger one. I ask the younger one to look after the older one,' comments Penny, mother of 11-year-old Barbara, who suffers developmental delay as well as epilepsy.

Grandparents

People of an older generation may be more prone to misunderstanding about epilepsy. They may still retain outdated ideas of social stigma, simply lack any knowledge of what epilepsy involves or be afraid of it. You may find that support from other families with epilepsy becomes more important, and you can meet these through national support groups. But you can also try to educate grandparents about the condition – by explaining exactly what it is or inviting them to attend one of your child's medical appointments so that they can meet his doctor. Sometimes they may be afraid to take your child on outings or have him to stay in case they cannot cope with his epilepsy. This is understandable, but it may be helpful to explain exactly what to do in the event of a seizure, and to emphasize that all your child is likely to need afterwards is rest – no special treatment.

■ UNDERSTANDING EPILEPSY

Understanding epilepsy yourself puts you in a strong position to reassure and support your child. Being informed not only helps the whole family to come to terms with the condition, but has practical implications too, as everyone in the family should know what to do in the event of a seizure.

Every case is different, so you will need to talk to your child's own doctor and epilepsy specialist about his individual situation. Epilepsy support groups and organizations can also provide a great deal of information in the form of brochures, books and videos. In addition, they provide a valuable point of contact for meeting other people who have epilepsy in the family. And they often have telephone helplines staffed by people with access to specialist knowledge, who may be able to answer specific queries.

■ GETTING TO KNOW YOUR CHILD'S CONDITION

Epilepsy can be idiosyncratic. Stuart, for example, tended to have more attacks in winter, when he was prone to fever, and he was frequently hospitalized because his high temperature triggered seizures, while Natalie's mother realized that she tended to have more seizures when she was constipated (which is relatively common).

A seizure diary is an invaluable tool for helping recognize any pattern which might emerge around your child's seizures and identifying any regular triggers – for example if he tends to have seizures in certain situations such as classes he finds stressful, after eating particular foods or after a run of late nights. Not everyone finds that such a pattern does emerge, but some parents have been able to identify quite specific triggers, such as cough medicine or the fumes from certain paints, as well as getting a clearer idea of lifestyle issues such as how much sleep and stimulation their child needed.

You may even be asked to keep a diary by your doctor, as a way of studying the nature of your child's seizures better, and of monitoring the effect of any anti-epileptic drugs. Finally, keeping a diary provides a way of making your child aware of triggers and is a means of gradually handing over responsibility to him.

Predicting seizures

Some parents get to know their children's epilepsy very well – indeed, they sometimes develop a sixth sense about when they are building up to a seizure. They become familiar with certain typical mood patterns, often of depression or moodiness, which may last some days or hours and culminate in a seizure (prodrome). It is thought these mood patterns come from abnormal brain activity, which finally builds up to an actual seizure. Your child, however, may not be aware of any change in mood, or of its impact on those around him.

The University of Kansas Medical Center in the USA is one of several research centres working on a method to predict seizures. Their technique uses sophisticated technology to measure brain activity, separating signals into seizure and non-seizure components, using mathematics, digital processing of EEG signals and computer technology. But so far the research is experimental – it may still be several years before a device is actually available.

■ TALKING TO YOUR CHILD ABOUT EPILEPSY

Informing your child about epilepsy is very important. He may have no idea of the true nature of his condition because he is not conscious during the attacks.

How much you tell him depends on the individual child and

how much you think he is ready for. Generally, the younger a child is, the more likely he is to be contented with a brief explanation. At some point, though, the chances are that you will need to go into more detail. Realistic, factual explanations can short-circuit fears and fantasies which may be preying on his mind, or help him deal with half-understood hints from outsiders.

Bearing in mind your child's age, ability and understanding of the condition, you may find it useful to prepare a kind of 'lesson' on epilepsy for him, perhaps with props such as diagrams of the brain and seizure activity. Some epilepsy organizations have material which has been specially prepared for children. You might also want to involve your doctor or a counsellor to help explain the condition, either at an initial discussion or later, when your child may have absorbed the initial information and want to ask questions. He may need several explanations and discussions before he really understands the situation.

Points you may want to cover include:

- exactly what epilepsy is
- why it happens
- what happens in a seizure
- what a person looks like in a seizure – videos or pictures can help
- the reassurance that although some seizures may look dramatic, the vast majority are painless for the person involved and it is extremely rare for anyone to die during a seizure (it may be worth stating this openly if you suspect your child is harbouring secret fears about this issue)
- how to manage epilepsy in terms of drugs, diet and lifestyle
- what to say to other people (children and adults), both about epilepsy in general, and if a seizure occurs (it may be worth establishing from the start that others are often ill-informed about the condition)

You should also encourage discussion and questions – this is not going to be a one-way process and you might be surprised at what has been on your child's mind. Beth, aged four, wanted to know if brain cells had legs or wings: she apparently thought they were a type of insect!

◼ INVOLVING YOUR CHILD

Involving your child in the management of his epilepsy can help him come to terms with it, as well as avoiding being overprotective. For example, depending on his age and ability you could encourage him to:

- take responsibility for his own medication
- research epilepsy for himself via libraries, computer information resources and epilepsy associations
- be aware of his triggers, such as lack of sleep (so long as he does not become obsessive about them)
- deal with other practicalities, such as carrying snacks if he suffers more seizures when he is hungry
- think positively, by explaining that controlling emotions such as stress can actually affect the nature and number of attacks
- buld his own relationship with the doctor and ask questions for himself, on the grounds that treatment is more likely to be successful if it comes out of a partnership (he can prepare for appointments by writing down questions, or taking in written information (articles, booklets) about something he wants to know more about)

Discuss who he wants to tell about his epilepsy, and why this may be positive for him. Talking about the condition reduces the stress of living a 'secret life', and helps foster more open and equal relationships (hiding something about yourself dents people's confidence and does not help build close relationships). It may also have practical implications in that people will be more aware of what is going on if he does have a seizure, and may know what help to give.

▪ BUILDING CONFIDENCE

Unconditional love and acceptance is vital for all children if they are to develop that precious asset, confidence. Confidence is particularly important for a child with epilepsy. He needs to know that he is a unique individual who can deal with a variety of situations, and this means practical knowledge; he needs to be given the chance to have a go at things, not just theoretical encouragement.

No matter how much you love your child, it will not help him to be given a label of being unwell. Nor will it help if he is allowed to use epilepsy as an excuse for non-achievement or for getting out of activities without even trying. 'Be realistic, not restrictive,' advises the National Society for Epilepsy in the UK. Obviously this means that, like the rest of us, your child will sometimes come up against his limitations, but at least epilepsy will not have stopped him having a go.

Here are some guidelines for building confidence.

* Correct and honest information about epilepsy has been high-lighted by many studies as being one of the most important factors in developing a child's self-esteem. Ensure that your child is a full partner in the management of his epilepsy, as described above, a concept which is rooted in respect for the child and can have a profound effect on his self-esteem.
* Do not make light of your child's problems, however trivial, cute or amusing they may seem.
* Confidence comes from success, feedback, activity and relationships – it does not exist in a vacuum. Get your child involved – in a sport, an activity or a club.
* Allow your child to experiment, become frustrated, make mistakes and even experience failure. Even if he aims too high, he will have the memory of the experience, and of exploring his own ability and resources. So trust your child and give him as much independence as possible. Do not be too quick to rescue or help him. Explain that failure is a risk

everyone takes when trying out some activities, but that it can be fun and worthwhile just having a go.

- Do not allow yourself to be frightened of exercising proper discipline by the possibility of a seizure. Your child will feel more secure, and so more confident, if he knows he has a steady and reliable parent behind him.

- Back up your endeavours with sensible safety precautions appropriate to your child's age and ability, and the nature of his epilepsy, such as cooker guards if he wants to cook. (Full advice on safety is available from epilepsy organizations – see 'Useful Adddresses'.)

- Encourage your child's social efforts, from casual conversations in the street to inviting a friend home for tea. Clubs and sports can teach him how useful a common interest is for forming relationships – a social skill which will help him well into adult life.

- Having high expectations for your child is a key factor, as he is likely to try to live up to them. However, it is also important that you accept him for what he is – a realistic acknowledgement of areas of weakness can make for more confidence if you give him the resources and support to meet any difficulties. For example, you could help him work out strategies for overcoming memory problems, such as using drug wallets, diaries and wall-charts.

ACTIVITIES AND EXERCISE

It is important to realize that many children with epilepsy can have perfectly normal childhoods and participate fully in activities and games, and there may be no need to restrict your family life. Some parents forbid certain activities for fear that their child will have a seizure during them, causing injury to themselves and others. But many doctors feel that the social and psychological damage done by restricting a child's life often probably outweighs the risks involved in many activities – excessive restriction and under-achievement have been described as common secondary handicaps of epilepsy, perhaps because this is society's and parents' way of managing the unmanageable.

In fact, research has shown that people are less likely to have a seizure when enjoyably occupied than when sitting alone on the sidelines, feeling bored and excluded and perhaps churning inside. Another point to remember is that although injuries can occur as a result of seizures, they are rare.

Exercise, which is vital in a society where increasing numbers of children are unfit and obese, has added relevance for a child with epilepsy, because by improving general fitness, stress levels and wellbeing, it reduces the likelihood of seizures. It also improves your child's general confidence and self-esteem and, in the case of team sports, gives him valuable opportunities for participating and sharing.

Children with epilepsy cannot be considered as a homogeneous group, and decisions about the type of activity which would best suit your child need to be made on an individual basis, taking the following into account:

- **how well controlled your child's seizures are**. Each child's epilepsy is different, and levels of control vary.
- **the risks of the particular activity**. Obviously some high-risk activities, such as scuba diving and rock climbing, will need extra consideration. It has to be remembered that in practical terms this may be an unusual occurrence (how many children actually go scuba diving at all, let alone regularly?). Likewise, precautions are sensible in certain activities such as swimming, but this applies to all children – no parent encourages a child to swim straight out to sea or to scale a sheer cliff face without proper preparation and supervision.
- **any extra supervision or precautions your child may need**. This may sometimes be the factor which tips the scales when deciding on an activity. Activity leaders should know about your child's epilepsy, and you then have a chance to see what, if anything, is on offer in terms of extra help.

Swimming is a very common case in point. An ideal form of exercise, it often raises fears and confusion in parents, teachers and swimming organizations because of safety concerns, although in fact research shows that few seizures happen in the water. Swimming is vital for safety – a child may be more likely to drown because he cannot swim than because he has a seizure in the water. Some parents have found they have to offer the extra supervision themselves, for example by attending school swimming classes with their children.

Sport – do doctors play it too safe?
Family doctors may be erring on the side of caution when it comes to advice on sport for people with epilepsy, according to a German study. In a series of fitness tests, including a 2 km walk, tests of muscle strength and aerobic tests, those with epilepsy had lower fitness levels than the control group. The study concludes that lower fitness levels affect general wellbeing, which can in turn affect seizure control. Health professionals should be educated in the advantages of people with epilepsy taking part in suitable physical fitness activities, the study concluded.

BEHAVIOUR PROBLEMS

Case Study
Michael found that he could trigger seizures by hyperventilating, something he did not hesitate to use to his own advantage, for example when asked to do something he did not want to do – and something which singularly failed to impress his mother, Jules!

Children are children, and behaviour problems are endemic in family life, whether epilepsy is present or not. Medical papers of the 19th century (and even some in the 20th century) are full of the idea of a special 'epileptic personality', but modern opinion is that this belongs firmly in the realm of myth. Children do not misbehave in seizures, though a child in post-ictal con-fusion (ie after a seizure) may hit out rather randomly if restrained or threatened.

Many children go through a difficult spell as a reaction to being diagnosed with epilepsy. They may have unstated fears and anxieties which show in behaviour rather than in verbal discussion, for example sleep disturbance, aggression towards other children, disobedience and regression such as bed-wetting. It may be a relief to your child if you try to bring his troubles out into the open – it may be something which seems insignificant to you, but which has immense significance to him. Stuart, for example, was bothered by a foreign voluntary helper at school who had some idiosyncratic term for epilepsy which he feared was an insult or put-down – a simple case of misunderstanding. It may also help to discuss the problem with teachers, the school nurse, your family doctor or school meals staff, whom some children regard as all-powerful!

There are some special causes of misbehaviour which can affect some children with epilepsy:

- the simple fact of having epilepsy, especially if seizures are frequent or it provokes bullying or teasing
- sub-clinical abnormal brain activity, which is not enough to produce a seizure but is enough to affect behaviour
- the side-effects of drugs, especially if the dose is too high

Epilepsy can have a behavioural and emotional component in that some children's seizures are made worse by stress, emotional upset or boredom. There may also be genuine frustration at having to miss out on opportunities, such as outings or hobbies, which their friends can enjoy without a thought. Missed absence seizures may also leave a child confused and frustrated. And it must not be overlooked that children's behaviour may go through upheavals because of their developmental timetable, the main example being adolescence.

Behaviour and learning disability

Behaviour is a key issue in the care of people with learning disability and epilepsy, according to a British epilepsy survey by Dr Michael Kerr and Stuart Todd, from the Welsh Centre for Learning Difficulties, Cardiff. 'The connection between behavioural problems and epilepsy is one which, as a parent, causes a great deal of distress: it is a problem which seems to be overlooked,' commented a carer. According to the survey, behavioural disturbance can take many different forms, from physical self-abuse to overt aggression, and the problem for carers such as parents is deciding what is causing the behaviour. The survey gives clues as to how to spot the three different causes for misbehaviour.

1 Behaviour caused by seizures. Clues may be:

• nothing obvious in the vicinity to cause your child to behave in that way
• the same behaviour each time
• confusion, drowsiness or a need for sleep around the same time
• typical behaviour patterns just before or after seizures

2 Behaviour caused by medication. Clues may be:

• the behaviour coinciding with a change in medication or dosage
• your child being too drowsy or too active between episodes of bad behaviour
• your child being off his food
• your child not sleeping well, or going through changes in sleep patterns
• uncharacteristic behaviour or longstanding behavioural problems which seem to be persisting or getting worse

3 Behaviour independent of seizures or medication. Clues may be:

• behaviour unrelated to seizures or medication
• behaviour as a constant problem

- the fact that changes in medication or the number of seizures seem to have no effect on the behaviour
- a suspicion that the behaviour may be the child's non-verbal way of asking for something or trying to avoid something

Who can help: your family doctor, a specialist nurse, an epilepsy specialist, local therapy and counselling resources.

HELPING YOUR CHILD COPE WITH STRESS

The link between stress and seizures is well established, and teaching your child to deal with stress is one of the most valuable ways you can help, both now and for the future. This avoids a dynamic of dependence on you and other authority figures such as teachers, or a vicious circle where the family or school is struggling to protect him from stress. Learning to deal with epilepsy and any associated stresses can make your child a stronger person for life.

Getting the right mental attitude involves some help from parents, who need to encourage positive thinking in whatever way they can. It helps too to make sure your child understands his epilepsy as far as possible – confusion is stressful. Above all, it is vital to learn to manage stress, not avoid it, and your child may need to learn that working through fear forms a part of stress management. For example, it is potentially stressful for any child, or even an adult, to walk into a strange class, find a place to sit, and start establishing relationships with those around him. Teaching your child to go through this kind of social pain barrier paves the way for the rewards of being relaxed and confident. On a social note also, your child may need to know how to stand up for himself and be assertive, which means developing good communication skills, and learning to relax.

Helping your child learn what it feels like to be relaxed is invaluable in stress management. Some of the complementary therapies covered in chapter 4 focus on relaxation; in addition, you might like to try massage, which is covered in chapter 5.

Otherwise, there is a wide variety of ways you can help your child relax – but bear in mind that children tend not to be very interested in relaxing if it means lying down doing nothing! Relaxation in children may be better defined as being quietly and enjoyably occupied, or as a contented state of mind. Here are some ways in which you can help your child manage stress.

- **Exercise**. The importance of fitness has already been discussed, and there is a wide range of stress-beating exercises available. Swimming is one of the best, and perhaps you might like to go too and share the benefits! Traditional team sports such as football usually focus on participation, sharing and self-discipline, benefits which fuel self-confidence and personality development. Other activities such as yoga (*see* chapter 4) or aikido or t'ai chi, are rooted in philosophies which may be very helpful in teaching your child to deal with personal and external stresses. T'ai chi, for example, is a martial art which focuses on relaxation, concentration and balance, and can be used for healing, self-defence, personal development and spiritual discipline. Class leaders should be informed about your child's epilepsy.
- **Art or music therapy**. Both these therapies help children express their feelings without the use of words, which can be deeply therapeutic for those who have not yet learned how to manage and manipulate words with adult skill. Look round for local art or music classes, or contact a national music therapy association for details (*see* 'Useful Addresses').
- **Diet**. This may be worth checking as the wrong sort can contribute to stress in different ways. For example, too much adrenalin, which is released when we are under stress, can deplete our store of certain vitamins, especially C and some B vitamins. This in turn can contribute to stress on the nervous system and generally lowered physical and mental resistance. Some children, especially teenagers, also eat differently when stressed, in particular 'comfort eating' or bingeing on sweets and chocolate, which may stress the body, tip the

balance of nutrients and perhaps lead to a seizure. In addition, allergies and intolerances can affect your child's emotional and mental state, which may be significant given the importance of an even emotional keel. See the section on nutrition below; chapter 4 gives information on nutritional therapy.

■ COPING WITH STRESS FOR PARENTS

Case Studies
'I make sure I go down to the pub one evening a week with my husband. We sit there and have a moan about Max – try and have a laugh about him and his antics. That helps us keep it all in proportion.'

'I burn fragrant aromatherapy oils in burners round the house, which I think is soothing for the whole family.'

'I'd say, be open about the epilepsy – trying to keep things secret and hidden is stressful.'

'I go to a local epilepsy support group where there's a lot of mums like me. We're managing – and that's something when it gets as difficult as it can do.'

Parenting is a hard job at the best of times, and it can be all too easy to overlook the fact that you need time to yourself. However, it is vital that you relax and make time for simple luxuries such as a relaxing bath, having half an hour alone with a cup of tea and a magazine, or chatting on the phone to a friend.

In addition, there may be times when you might feel the need for something more in your life, something special – when the stress really piles up, when you go through a long run of difficulties or depression, when life seems grey, or you want to create a new mood. You may also need help coping with emotions which can have added force when you are dealing with a condition such as epilepsy, questions like guilt, anxiety and anger, and balancing your deep urge to protect your child with the equal necessity of letting him go.

You might be tempted to dismiss some of the techniques suggested below as luxuries, for which you have no time or money. However, while some stress may get the adrenalin going and help spur you into action, too much is counterproductive and makes you increasingly less effective. Stress reduces your resistance and can make you ill. If you allow it to build up too much, not only will you be less able to meet the demands of your child, your family and the rest of your life, but it will also have a knock-on effect on your child. Moreover, children learn from example, and setting a good example of stress management can be extremely helpful for your child, who may well find that coping with stress is the key to management of his epilepsy in both childhood and adulthood. Given the particular risk of low self-esteem in epilepsy, it can only help your child if he sees you enhance your own self-esteem. The following are only suggestions, and you will find many more in good books on reducing stress (*see* 'Further Reading').

▓ De-stressing the body

Stress is felt in the body as much as in the mind, so you need ways to let go of physical stress. Massage can be an enjoyable way to do this, perhaps with aromatherapy oils. Relaxing oils include cedarwood, chamomile, clary sage, juniper berry, lavender, mandarin, marjoram, mimosa, myrrh, sandalwood, valerian, vetiver, violet leaf and ylang ylang. (But avoid chamomile and clary sage during pregnancy, and if you want to try aromatherapy massage on your child, see pages 96–7, especially the warning about which oils are contra-indicated in epilepsy.)

Skin bathing may conjure up visions of a 19th-century spa, but it has always been popular on the continent as a healthy way of airing the body and boosting wellbeing, so try spending a quarter of an hour or so unclothed, outside if possible – weather permitting! Dry skin brushing is another natural cure method, which involves gently brushing the skin with a vegetable bristle brush as a means of stimulating the circulation and elimination processes, among other benefits.

Forty minutes in a flotation tank is supposed to be worth six hours of sleep, and this therapy is also said to aid meditation as well as relaxation. It involves lying in a completely dark tank of salt water at body temperature, so that external stimuli are blocked out. Some people find this claustrophobic or just boring, but if you are desperately busy and tired, it can be highly relaxing to be in a position where you are forced to do nothing.

Physical exercise is another proven de-stressor. If you really are too busy to fit in an exercise class or a visit to the swimming pool, simply leaving the car behind and walking briskly will help revitalize you. Keeping in tune with the daily weather changes can be soothing, and the physical movement stimulates your circulation, improves fitness and helps release endorphins, the body's natural opiates. This is of course also true of more structured exercise, such as yoga, which works on the mind and emotions as well as the body, and incorporates breathing exercises, which are very important in overall wellbeing. Or it could be a matter of taking up an activity which gets you right out of the house and into another world for a couple of hours – one mother took up riding every Saturday afternoon, while another couple built a session at the local bowling alley into their week.

De-stressing your mind and spirit

Meditation can involve simply having time to yourself, or spending a few minutes looking out at the moon or attending to changes in the weather or seasons. Or it can be a more directed ten minutes taken out to sit quietly, focusing on your breathing or on an object such as a candle. Some people may benefit from combining meditation with another remedy such as flower remedies, which are believed to work on your energy, emotions and spirit (*see* chapter 4).

Healing sounds can also be used as meditation aids, or on their own as a relaxation technique. Many people find natural sounds such as rain and thunder soothing, and these are available on cassettes. Music also remains a time-honoured way of helping you create your own inner space or personal sanctuary. The human heart beats at a rate of 70–80 beats a minute, so that any music with a rhythm of less than 80 beats a minute is perceived as slow and relaxing as it works on the brain's limbic system, which is involved in emotions and instinctive responses.

A healing environment

The effect of colour on mood has been well documented, and while you may not want to plunge into major redecoration, you can create subtle but enhancing changes with accessories such as cushions and rugs. Relaxing colours are blue, indigo and violet; warm, healing colours include gold, orange, peach and cream.

Feng shui is the ancient Chinese art of placement, and means arranging homes so as to facilitate the flow of qi (chi) or life energy through them (qi is explained more fully in chapter 4). If the life force is blocked by too much clutter or the incorrect placement of objects in the home, the result can be poor health and unhappiness, according to feng shui sages. Feng shui does not have to be elaborate – it could just be a matter of clearing out all the old clothes and outworn toys, and adding one or two carefully chosen items such as plants, wind chimes and mirrors, which in feng shui play an important part in redirecting qi and can be placed so as to add light and dimension to a room.

Getting help

In addition to contacting an epilepsy support group, you may also feel the need for more personal reassurance and perhaps spiritual or emotional guidance. Help from others can take many forms. On one level, for example, a spiritual healer can work with you to deal better with any negative forces blocking your energy and happiness, or perhaps to help you let go of any compulsion to control an uncontrollable situation and to create more acceptance. Hypnotherapy induces a state of deep relaxation in which you can clear away negative thoughts and unconscious worries, have a better look at problems, and work out strategies for dealing with them.

These days, there are so many people offering 'intuitive healing', 'spiritual guidance' and the like that it can be very hard to know which to choose. A good starting point is something or someone you feel intuitively drawn to, or someone who comes recommended by a friend. Bear in mind that it may take a bit of trial and error to find the right person for you, so do not hesitate to move on if you feel uncomfortable with your initial choice.

More directly practical outside help may also be available, depending on where you live. This may include medical care, advice, information and counselling, day care, after-school and holiday provision, help with transport and holidays, cultural, social and leisure activities, short-term or respite care and much more. Above all, do not forget the epilepsy organizations – many parents have found these invaluable as a source of support.

◾ NUTRITION

The whole family benefits from following a healthy diet, which lessens stress, builds up resistance to illness and makes for more mental balance. Basic healthy eating rules include: keeping to a low-fat, low-sugar diet with plenty of fresh fruit and vegetables; eating whole foods such as wholewheat bread and brown rice; avoiding processed and refined foods; and eating a variety of foods. The suggestions below for keeping blood sugar levels steady can also form part of a healthy eating plan. And, if you do feel you need to make reforms, it is best to introduce changes gradually, over a few weeks or months.

Some children with epilepsy may suffer food allergies or

intolerance or some form of nutritional imbalance. These problems are dealt with in chapter 4.

▪ Keeping your child's blood sugar level steady

This can be a family issue, but it may have particular relevance for children with epilepsy, as low blood sugar (hypoglycaemia) has been noted as a common accompaniment to seizures; mood swings are also a common sign of low blood sugar in some children with epilepsy. Moreover, keeping blood sugar levels steady may be particularly important for teenage girls, to help them avoid mood dips before their periods. Paying attention to blood sugar level can also help parents – the 'quick fix' of a coffee and biscuit is a notorious source of stress.

Proper nutrition helps in this. Basically, when you eat, glucose from the food passes through your intestine into the bloodstream, where your body uses it for energy. If the glucose level rises too high, the pancreas tends to flood the body with insulin to lower it. This may result in low blood sugar symptoms such as fatigue, irritability and the craving for more sugary foods. This can throw your body into confusion, impacting on the adrenal glands, which then work harder, so further exacerbating stress. The following will help maintain balanced blood sugar levels for your child and the whole family.

- Make sure the whole family has breakfast – porridge, unsugared muesli, wholemeal toast, poached egg, etc.
- Try to ensure that your child has a regular food intake, with healthy snacks every two or three hours to bridge the gap between meals. Snacks do not have to be huge – carrot sticks, fruit, dried fruit such as figs or scones or biscuits made with wholemeal flour are ideal.
- Cut down on all sources of sugar – chocolate, sweets, cakes, biscuits – as well as sugary drinks such as fizzy drinks and squash.
- Also cut down on refined foods such as white flour and

breakfast cereals, and processed foods in tins and packets such as tinned pasta or packet soup.

- Eat unrefined complex carbohydrates such as wholemeal bread, wholemeal pasta, potatoes, brown rice, beans, lentils, chickpeas, nuts or seeds.

Mood foods

'Make your food your medicine' is the age-old advice from Hippocrates – but can foods really affect your mood or even cure the brain? Nutritional therapists at the Institute for Optimum Nutrition, London (ION) think the right nutrients can help the brain rebalance its own chemistry. The Director of the ION, Patrick Holford, believes that certain nutrients can help a wide range of emotional and mental imbalances such as learning difficulty.

Suggested nutrients for a positive outlook, and which may help the mood swings from which many children with epilepsy suffer, include:

- **Vitamin B complex.** These vitamins are needed for the smooth running of the central nervous system. They help improve blood flow throughout the body, so ensuring that the brain is well supplied with oxygen. Sources include wholegrain products, egg yolks, fish, nuts, beans, tofu, cheese, brewer's yeast and yoghurt.
- **Vitamin C.** This helps your body beat stress. It is found in citrus fruits, blackcurrants, broccoli and all fresh fruit and vegetables.
- **Magnesium.** A lack causes irritability, nervousness and depression. It is found in dairy foods, meat and seafood.
- **Manganese.** This works with B vitamins to ensure a healthy nervous system, and is found in avocados, nuts, seeds, wholegrain products, egg yolks and pineapples.
- **Zinc.** This helps the immune system function, and a lack can cause problems such as mental lethargy and sluggish sex glands. It is found in pumpkin seeds, nuts, wholegrain oysters, brewer's yeast, egg yolks, meat and poultry.

■ WHAT TO DO IN THE EVENT OF A SEIZURE

Attacks cannot be stopped, so do not try to restrain your child during a seizure, or let other people interfere, crowd round or try to touch him.

■ Convulsive seizures

- Put something soft under your child's head and only move him if he is in danger (eg in the road).
- Do not put anything in his mouth.
- Once convulsions have stopped, roll your child onto his side, into the recovery position.
- Wipe away any saliva, and if your child is still breathing with difficulty check that there is nothing in his mouth, such as food.
- Stay with your child to help reassure him until he feels able to get on with what he was doing, or take him home to rest.

■ Non-convulsive seizures

These seizures vary and may need different responses. In prolonged confusion:

- Gently guide your child away from obvious dangers such as traffic.
- Speak calmly and gently to him to help him reorientate himself.
- Stay with your child until he is able to resume what he was doing. Bear in mind that he may be confused for some time after the attack, and because of this may sound aggressive, so it may be best to stay fairly quiet until he has come round.

Get medical help if:

- a seizure lasts longer than five minutes and you do not know how long they usually last
- your child has trouble breathing after a seizure
- he has hurt himself badly during a seizure

Chapter Three

Conventional Treatments

A skilled epilepsy team can make all the difference to your child's life but, in addition, both you and she can play a vital role in treatment. Traditionally, doctors have tended to treat epilepsy by treating seizures – in other words, by suppressing them with drugs. Vital as this is, there is now more emphasis on quality of life, and increasing recognition that the best treatment for each child is one which is arrived at by medical carers working in partnership with families (even if for some parents this is an ideal rather than a reality at present).

Given that around 75–80 per cent of children have their seizures controlled by drugs, medication remains the main form of treatment you will be considering. Your heart may sink at the thought of your child having to take drugs on a long-term basis. You may worry about the fact that they are unnatural, wonder whether they are mind altering, or be concerned that they will make her dopey or drag her down. Generally, the more modern drugs work more efficiently and have fewer-side effects than old ones, but their impact on your child does have to be monitored, again on an individual basis. Your epilepsy specialist will work to ensure that your child has the type and dose of drug which suits her best, and this can vary a good deal from child to child, depending on the nature of her epilepsy, and how her metabolism processes drugs. On the positive side, eight out of ten children can achieve good seizure control with medication – and, since many children outgrow their epilepsy, drug treatment need not necessarily be for life. In addition, complementary therapies may have a part to play in helping achieve drug reduction, provided this is done cautiously and *only* under the guidance of a competent physician. Some parents have found that they have been able to reduce prescribed medication by arranging complementary treatment. As every child is different, this is something which needs individual discussion with both your complementary and your conventional pracitioner, and there is no reason why practitioners from both disciplines should not meet together to discuss how their respective treatments may overlap, and whether drug reduction is possible. Many reputable alternative practitioners are only too happy to do this.

■ THE PROBLEMS OF DIAGNOSIS

Case Studies
'Charlie's had blood tests, EEG, which didn't show anything, and MRI [Magnetic Resonance Imaging], which showed his brain was fine,' says his mother, Jane. 'At one point they thought it might be Landau–Kleffner syndrome, but that seems to have gone by the board. We haven't really got a diagnosis. It's complicated because his epilepsy is incidental to his development problems. It's only when you start investigating that you realize how very little the doctors do sometimes know.'

Jules, mother of Michael, aged 12, says: 'Michael has temporal lobe epilepsy, one of the more common kinds, which starts from a certain part of the brain. It took us about four years to get that diagnosis, though we now realize he must have had epilepsy well before that – we just didn't spot it, partly because his development and abilities are normal for his age.'

Diagnosing epilepsy is fraught with uncertainty. We tend to believe that doctors know everything and will hand out a neat medical label which will explain what we've 'got'. But, it can take months, or even years, to obtain a diagnosis of epilepsy. There may be repeated referrals, which can be very draining for families who may be impatient for a clear-cut medical decision, or who may feel that doctors are passing the buck by submitting the child to yet another investigation. Delays waiting for appointments, and overworked epilepsy clinics, do not help either.

But if getting a diagnosis is frustrating for parents, it is not always straightforward for doctors either, and there are reasons why it can take time to get a definitive diagnosis. First, if in doubt, many doctors tend not to diagnose epilepsy because of the potential impact on a child's life. Not only does it probably mean starting a long-term course of medication, it also has serious implications for education, social life and general health and wellbeing. So a definitive diagnosis may be deferred until they can be sure beyond reasonable doubt that a child does have epilepsy. This may be further complicated by the fact that epilepsy often does not have a single, obvious cause – no reason for the condition can be discovered in more than two-thirds of children.

In addition, there are many other disorders which may resemble epilepsy, and which can be misdiagnosed as epilepsy (*see* pages 15–18). Moreover, seizures may sometimes be just part of a complex picture of developmental delay or other problems, so that it may be hard even for epilepsy experts to decide on the precise type involved. To complicate matters further, there are several different types of epilepsy, and of epilepsy syndromes, so that again it may take time to decide exactly what a child has.

There is also no one test which can tell definitively if someone has epilepsy or not – the way a blood test can detect anaemia, for example – and repeated medical investigations may be necessary before treatment can be started.

■ MEDICAL HISTORY

So, how do doctors go about detecting epilepsy? This is one area where parents play a key part in helping the doctor make a diagnosis. This is because your doctor relies very much on eye-witness accounts of what actually happens during a seizure. Unless your child has another attack while actually with the doctor, the doctor will not have a clear idea of what happens, and what type of seizure is involved. An observer's description can be crucial in helping decide what sort of epilepsy, if any, is present.

For this reason, your doctor will not only want a detailed medical history of your child from babyhood, but will ask you several questions about the attack, such as what time of day it took place, how long it lasted and what exactly your child did during it – for example, fell limply, rolled her eyes or started jerking. Your doctor may also want to know (if you can remember) what your child was doing just before the attack and whether she seemed to have any particular symptoms such as depression, vagueness, nausea or pallor. Finally, you may be asked how your child behaved afterwards, whether she seemed confused, and how long it took to recover.

If epilepsy is suspected, your doctor should refer your child for further tests.

■ DIAGNOSTIC TESTS

■ Electroencephalogram (EEG)

As well as confirming your child's medical history, hospital specialists will arrange other tests for epilepsy. The most common one is electroencephalography (EEG), which examines how the brain behaves, and can differentiate normal from abnormal brainwave patterns.

This test measures the electrical activity of your child's brain cells, using electrodes which are placed on the scalp, and this activity is printed out and analysed to see if it shows epileptic patterns. About 12 electrodes are used in babies, and 20 in older children and teenagers, and although it may be distressing to see your child 'wired up' in this way the main discomfort actually appears to be in trying to wash the adhesive out afterwards!

The limitation of EEGs is that they often appear normal between seizures, so it may still be unclear whether your child has epilepsy. Equally, EEGs may show epileptic patterns between seizures, and some people who have never had seizures may show epileptic activity on an EEG. Doctors will therefore not diagnose epilepsy just on the basis of an abnormal EEG reading. Brain patterns also vary according to age – in the early years, up to around age seven or eight, the brain is developing rapidly, and in general, adult EEG patterns are reached by around 10–12.

To obtain a clearer result, doctors may ask you to ensure that your child has less sleep than usual before the test, as sleep deprivation can trigger abnormal brain activity. Alternatively, some EEGs may be done during sleep, either natural or drug-induced, as some abnormal brain patterns show up more clearly during sleep. In the course of the test, your child may also be asked to open and close her eyes, to breathe deeply and to look at a flashing light – all mechanisms which can trigger epileptic activity.

There are other tests which make use of EEG in a slightly different way. *EEG ambulatory monitoring* is EEG monitoring over a period of several hours. Your child will have EEG electrodes fixed onto her head, but will be allowed to leave the hospital and go home to carry on with her usual activities. The electrodes are attached to a small tape recorder, which records the brain waves. Because monitoring lasts longer, it is much more likely to pick up abnormal activity or a seizure. The tape is then returned to hospital for analysis. At some centres, EEG is also combined with video investigation, while the child stays in hospital for a day or more. This is called *video telemetry*. EEG monitoring takes place while a video camera records any seizures, and EEG patterns can then be analysed to help decide which type of epilepsy your child has. Obviously, this is more practicable in a child who has frequent seizures, but it may also pick up some abnormal activity between seizures.

Brain scans

Brain scans are the other main form of testing for epilepsy, but they are not performed routinely. Scans look at the overall make-up of the brain, and detect abnormalities which might be causing the epilepsy. Children are therefore more likely to be referred for scans if doctors suspect that there might be something amiss with their brain structure, which does not apply to every child. (The newer scans look at how the brain is working, too, but tend not to be widely available.) Referral for a scan can be daunting, and it can also be frustrating. Just when you think this will be the test to provide the answer, the scan may give a 'normal' reading. The fact is that, as already mentioned, the reasons for epilepsy cannot always be found, even by the most sophisticated scanning techniques.

Computerized axial tomography (CT or CAT) is a specialized type of X-ray, which can show the more obvious sort of brain damage or abnormality, such as congenital malformation (ie when the brain has not developed properly). Your child will have to lie still on a table for 15–20 minutes (she may be given a light sedative if necessary), while a rotating X-ray machine takes pictures of the brain from different angles. Several tiny, narrow beams of radiation pass through the brain at different levels, providing pictures of cross-sections or 'slices' of the brain. These pictures are then analysed by computer. If the initial pictures seem to show up something, a special dye is injected via the hand or arm, which shows the image more clearly on the scan.

Magnetic Resonance Imaging (MRI) is a much more sophisticated scanning technique which measures the energy given out by hydrogen atoms within the brain and then creates a picture based on these signals. By bouncing magnetic fields and radio waves (not radiation) off the brain, it forms very detailed pictures of the brain structure. Whereas previously epilepsy might have been written off as idiopathic (of unknown cause), MRI may now sometimes be able to pinpoint subtle abnormalities which older forms of investigation may have missed, such as minor congenital malformations of the brain which may cause epilepsy. Its precision also makes it particularly useful as a pre-surgery test (*see* pages 71–2). The test usually takes around 45 minutes and involves lying in a kind of tunnel while pictures are taken – a procedure some children may find frightening as well as noisy. Again, a light anaesthetic can help.

There are two newer types of scan which show how the brain is actually performing, as well as giving pictures of its underlying structure. In a few research centres, *Positron Emission Tomography (PET)* imaging is used to identify areas of the brain which are producing seizures. The images come from radioactive chemicals which are injected into the body and reach the brain, where they concentrate, so showing up specific areas more clearly. *Single Photon Emission Computerized Tomography (SPECT)* works on the same principle and may take over from it as a more efficient testing tool to show up seizure sources (areas of the brain from which seizures start).

▓ Other tests

Blood tests are done to check for any underlying disease which might be causing seizures, and to check the health of organs such as the liver and kidneys. They can also give information about possible vitamin deficiencies, any toxins in the blood and chemical abnormalities which could be causing seizures, especially in tiny babies. A lumbar puncture may be carried out if it is suspected that an infection such as encephalitis or meningitis is causing seizures. Finally, it is useful to have an idea of the state of a child's blood before starting anti-epileptic drugs, so that any changes made by the drugs will be more obvious in future blood tests.

Neuropsychological or neuropsychometric tests are simple tests which may be used to evaluate brain functions such as your child's memory, language and spatial perception. They may give clues as to precisely which type of epilepsy is affecting her or, occasionally, they may be used as pre-surgery tests.

■ STARTING TREATMENT

It may not always be in your child's best interests to be put straight onto drugs and, depending on the individual child, your doctor may decide on a wait-and-see approach. Most doctors would agree that a single seizure should not be treated with drugs, and that you should wait for at least two to occur. Again, the type of epilepsy may not need treating – seizures in BREC, for example, may be quite mild and happen only at night.

Depending on the nature of your child's epilepsy, your doctor – and you – may need to weigh up her overall need for drugs, which is different from an adult's. Children do not drive or operate machinery and may suffer less from the psycho-social impact of a seizure. Also, epilepsy in children is more likely to disappear of its own accord (spontaneous remission) than in adults. Moreover, the side-effects of some anti-epileptic drugs on your child's thinking powers and behaviour may be more insidious at a vulnerable age, and at a key time in her emotional and academic development. However, all this needs to be weighed up against the disabling effect of continuing seizures.

Many doctors believe that treatment for epilepsy should be started sooner rather than later because it achieves better control and makes for a better prognosis generally. There is some evidence to show that delaying treatment may make epilepsy worse, and could make control harder to achieve later on, so treatment is generally started after two seizures. However, other research suggests that treatment could be delayed longer to see if it is really needed. Work in Holland found that, among more than 200 children whose treatment was delayed until they had had four seizures, 40 per cent became seizure-free without drugs, while an estimated 50 per cent of children who have had a first tonic–clonic seizure, and no underlying disease, will not have another within two years.

Finally, treatment involves far more than just giving out drugs. Ideally, your doctor should be able to offer counselling on broader issues such as the general management of epilepsy and safety issues. Some practices or clinics may be able to offer contact with a specially trained epilepsy liaison nurse.

■ WHICH DRUG?

Once the decision to treat has been made, your doctor will decide on the drug of first choice. Doctors usually prefer to try just one drug (monotherapy) to start with. The choice will be based on:

- the type of seizures
- your child's age
- how well the drug works (its efficacy)
- possible side-effects

The aim of drug treatment is to control seizures with minimal side-effects, and doctors usually start at a lower dose and build up, in order to avoid side-effects as much as possible. Curiously, it is not known exactly how some of the established anti-epileptic drugs work, but they are thought to slow down the tendency of brain cells to fire, or to alter brain chemicals so as to achieve a better balance of electrical activity.

Steroids are occasionally prescribed for some difficult-to-treat epilepsy in the form of corticosteroids. These do not always work and have potentially serious side-effects, such as high blood pressure, a reduction in the body's immunity and weight gain.

Regular monitoring is obviously important to keep assessing

the effect of drugs in your growing child as her weight changes, particularly in adolesence. Your doctor may perform blood tests to check drug levels, although this is done more with some drugs than others, as some do not show up reliably in the blood.

Side-effects

Behaviour, moodiness and concentration are areas which commonly create anxiety among parents when their children are put on drugs. Some drugs do affect behaviour, especially at first and if the dose is too high, so it is worth discussing this with your doctor, who may be able to adjust the dosage.

Typical dose-related side-effects include drowsiness, lethargy, dizziness, unsteadiness or a skin rash. These should be discussed with your doctor as soon as possible. Side-effects may pass off with time as your child becomes accustomed to the drug, but should always be mentioned to your doctor. A few side-effects are serious, affecting the skin, liver and bone marrow, but this is very rare.

Older drugs, such as phenobarbitone and phenytoin (in use before the Second World War) tend to have more side-effects and may affect your child's behaviour and learning ability. Typical are problems with memory, alertness and concentration, as well as irritability and hyperactivity. For this reason they are less often prescribed. Newer drugs such as carbamazepine and sodium valproate (first used in the 1960s and 1970s) have fewer side-effects and the latest drugs such as vigabatrin, piracetam, gabapentin and topiramate are targeted more specifically at epilepsy, and may have even fewer side-effects, although possible long-term side-effects may not yet have been established.

The section on the main anti-epileptic drugs below should be treated as a general guideline only – consult your doctor for more information.

■ **First-line drugs** (Your doctor may try the following first, usually one at a time.)

- **Carbamazepine**

Used for: generalized tonic–clonic and partial seizures

Side-effects: possible skin rash, double vision, dizziness, unsteadiness, confused thinking and nausea initially or if the dose is too high; possible drop in the white blood cells which help fight infection, although this usually is not serious, and may only be temporary; anaplastic anaemia, when the bone marrow stops producing blood cells – extremely rare but serious

- **Ethosuximide**

Used for: absence seizures

Side-effects: nausea, headache, drowsiness; very rarely, rash, blood problems and liver diseases

- **Lamotrigine** (not for under-16s)

Used for: partial and generalized tonic–clonic seizures

Side-effects: skin rash, Stevens–Johnson syndrome (a severe, potentially life-threatening rash), drowsiness, double vision, dizziness and headache

- **Phenytoin**

Used for: generalized tonic–clonic and partial seizures

Side-effects: possible skin rash, drowsiness, unsteadiness and slurred speech if the dose is too high; possible behavioural and learning problems; decreased energy and alertness; coarsening of facial features, increased body hair (hirsutism), gum overgrowth and acne with prolonged therapy; possible but rare effects on liver or bone marrrow

- **Sodium valproate**

Used for: generalized tonic–clonic, partial and absence seizures

Side-effects: drowsiness and tremor (infrequently); hair loss (which is reversible); very rarely, liver damage (for this reason, it is not recommended in very young children – severe, sometimes fatal, liver failure occurs in one out of every 800 children under two, one out of 7,000 between two and ten, and fewer than one in 100,000 older than ten); not for babies under a year

■ **Second-line drugs** (These are prescribed less often and usually in combination with other drugs.)

• **Acetazolomide**
Used for: generalized tonic–clonic, partial and atypical absence seizures
Side-effects: lack of appetite, loss of weight, drowsiness, depression, pins and needles in hands and feet, joint pains, increased urine output, thirst, headache, dizziness, fatigue, irritability

• **Clobazam**
Used for: generalized tonic–clonic and partial seizures
Side-effects: drowsiness

• **Clonazepam**
Used for: partial, absence and myoclonic seizures
Side-effects: drowsiness, sedation

• **Gabapentin**
Used for: partial seizures
Side-effects: drowsiness, dizziness, headache, fatigue

• **Phenobarbitone**
Used for: generalized tonic–clonic and partial seizures
Side-effects: drowsiness, sedation, mental slowness

• **Piracetam**
Used for: myoclonic seizures
Side-effects: very rare but may include weight gain, diarrhoea, insomnia, drowsiness, nervousness, depression and rash

• **Primidone**
Used for: generalized tonic–clonic and partial seizures
Side-effects: nausea, unsteadiness, drowsiness, sedation, mental slowness

• **Topiramate**
Used for: partial seizures
Side-effects: weight loss, ataxia, kidney stones, impaired concentration, confusion, dizziness, fatigue, pins and needles, drowsiness

• **Vigabatrin**
Used for: partial and secondary generalized seizures

Side-effects: drowsiness, nausea, behaviour and mood changes; psychotic reactions

▧ WHAT IF THE DRUGS DO NOT WORK?

If the drugs do not work, many doctors recommend that the regime be kept as simple as possible (rational therapy) – ie, prescribing no more than two drugs, or just trying a higher dose. Your doctor will be aiming to lessen the risk of side-effects and toxicity, and using more than two drugs increases the likelihood of side-effects, possibly without having much extra effect on seizures.

Some types of seizure are harder than others to control with drugs, including myoclonic, atonic, tonic and partial seizures. Syndromes which are difficult to control include West syndrome, Lennox–Gastaut syndrome and severe myoclonic syndrome.

It can take time to achieve the right type and dose of drug for your child – different children need different amounts of drugs, depending on individual factors such as their metabolism and build (a higher dose does not mean that the epilepsy is worse). Moreover, many epilepsy drugs take a while to work. This said, in around 20–25 per cent of cases, drug treatment just does not work, although around 5–10 per cent of children respond to a combination of two drugs.

▧ CAN YOUR CHILD STOP TAKING THE DRUGS?

It is usually recommended that your child stay on anti-epileptic medication for at least two years and, as with starting with drugs, both the risks and the benefits of withdrawal have to be weighed up. Drugs must only be stopped with the support and supervision of your doctor, who will reduce medication over a period of around six to eight weeks. The good news is that successful withdrawal of drugs is more likely in children than in people whose epilepsy begins in adulthood.

Parents can probably think of several reasons for withdrawing medication, not least the possible side-effects, the bother of having to take them every day, the constant reminder they bring of 'having epilepsy', and the risk of psychological dependence (some children only feel safe or confident when taking the drugs). Children have less to lose than adults in at least trying to withdraw, as they do not risk losing a job or their driving licence; and, if seizures do return, control can usually be re-established with medication again.

In some cases, doctors can make an informed guess as to whether seizures will return, but it remains impossible to give hard and fast predictions. Seizures do return in a little more than a third of children, but research has shown that some factors increase the risk of recurrence, including:

- a known cause for the epilepsy
- seizures starting after the age of 12
- a family history of epilepsy
- a history of atypical febrile seizures

If seizures do return, they normally do so relatively soon – in 50 per cent of cases within six months of stopping medication, in 60–80 per cent within a year, and in virtually all cases within two years. Careful planning may be required with older children and teenagers to make sure that a possible return of seizures does not interfere with examinations or learning to drive.

▨ DISAGREEING WITH TREATMENT

Case Study
Daniel only had seizures at night, but the family doctor insisted that he needed carbamazepine. His mother, Debbie, was very reluctant to put her son on heavy-duty drugs,

especially as she knew that treatment could last for several years.

If you do not agree with what your doctor has prescribed for your child, it is obviously best to discuss this with him or her face to face. If you still cannot agree, there are various options you can try.

- You can get a second opinion. You should inform your family doctor that you are doing this.
- You can contact a national epilepsy support group, who may be able to advise you on a specialist epilepsy centre. You can then ask your family doctor for a referral, although you will probably have to wait a while for an appointment.
- You can explore complementary therapies (*see* chapter 4), but again it is important that you tell your usual doctor, and vital that you do not suddenly withdraw your child from anti-epileptic drugs.

■ SURGERY

Epilepsy surgery has traditionally been viewed as only suitable for a minority of people whose condition has failed to respond to drug treatment. In the UK, for example, just 100–200 children, usually with intractable epilepsy, undergo surgery each year. However, it has been suggested that the number could be between 1,500 and 2,000 if there were sufficient proper facilities.

Over the past few years, however, there seems to have been a growing feeling that doctors have been over-cautious in prescribing surgery and, with new imaging and surgical techniques, more operations have been performed over the last decade or so.

You may well want to consider surgery if you are faced with the daily consequences of intractable epilepsy – the possibility of physical injury during seizures, the side-effects of a combination of drugs, the way seizures interfere with learning and disrupt family and social life, and worries about your child's quality of life and future development.

Surgery can be a safe and viable procedure for many children, and may even have specific advantages. A younger brain has more plasticity, and can relearn and reorganize better, so increasing the prospects of overall recovery. A successful operation which gets rid of epilepsy at a young age may also help avoid psycho-social and educational damage, making for better relationships with family and friends, and improving educational prospects.

When is surgery possible?

Doctors are highly conscious of the irreversible nature of surgery and approach it with great caution because of the risks involved. It is only done under very stringent conditions, which may vary in detail from centre to centre but tend to run along the following lines.

- The seizures must be disabling – that is, frequent and severe enough to interfere drastically with schooling and social or family life.
- The seizures should be medically intractable – that is, not respond to drug treatment.
- The seizures must start from a specific place in the brain, which can be pinpointed by investigative methods such as EEG, MRI and PET.
- Surgery must not be done in areas of the brain which involve essential functions such as language and memory.
- Families have to understand the risks as well as the benefits, and should be given information about both success rates and dangers.

How successful is surgery? Outcomes may vary from centre to centre, but, typically 60–75 per cent of operations have good outcomes, banishing seizures completely or reducing them substantially. The main risks have to do with strokes, causing paralysis and/or speech problems. Other risks include anaesthetic complication and infection – all potentially serious, capable of causing further brain damage and even death. Although these risks are rare, it is *your* child who is involved, not an anonymous figure from the statistics. You need plenty of time to weigh up all considerations, and to talk to your child's medical carers.

The decision whether to operate or not may only be arrived at after several months – or longer. It will be discussed by a variety of people at your child's hospital, involving for example adult and paediatric epileptologists, neurosurgeons, neuropsychologists, neuroradiologists, nurses and social workers. In addition, extensive tests will be performed before surgery is given the go-ahead, including:

- depth electrodes, which are fine silver needles, like normal electrodes but penetrating the brain, and which pick up the epileptic activity more precisely
- MRI spectroscopy, a refinement of MRI which measures metabolites, chemicals within the brain, and can pinpoint the site of lesions before surgery
- detailed neuropsychological tests to make sure that surgery will not affect vital brain areas by assessing language, memory, concentration, motor, visual-spatial and other skills – modern imaging methods are used

How surgery works

Epilepsy surgery in children currently takes two forms: *resective* and *disconnection surgery.* Resective surgery removes the source of the seizures, such as a scar or cyst. A team of specialists identifies the part of the brain which causes the child's seizures and then removes this epileptic zone.

Disconnective surgery disconnects the seizure source (the part of the brain from which seizures start) from other parts. This is done by cutting the nerve fibres so that seizure activity can no longer travel along the nerve pathways. In other words, it interferes with the spread of a seizure, but does not remove the part of the brain which causes a seizure.

▍ Types of operation

The most commonly performed operation for epilepsy is *temporal lobectomy*. This involves removing the part of the temporal lobe responsible for complex partial seizures, which may be tiny, measuring only a few centimetres.

Hemispherectomy (literally 'removal of a hemisphere') may be the best option for some children whose epilepsy involves one hemisphere of their brain, such as those with Sturge–Weber syndrome or Rasmussen's syndrome, when seizures are often hard to control with drugs. It sounds drastic, but once the poorly functioning section is removed, the remaining brain often compensates for the loss, especially with the plasticity of the childhood brain. Also, whereas years ago a complete hemisphere might have been removed, today's operation is much modified, often making use of specialized disconnection techniques as well as resective ones. In one common procedure, for example, *functional hemispherectomy*, the temporal lobe is removed, corpus callosotomy (*see* below) is performed, and the frontal and occipital lobes are disconnected. It is still major surgery, but it does leave the blood supply to the remaining brain intact, and the skull remains filled on the side of the operation rather than being left with a large gap.

The main type of disconnection surgery is a *corpus callosotomy* (or corpus callosum section), which involves the division of the corpus callosum, the large bundle of nerve fibres which passes electrical information from one hemisphere to the other and is the main pathway along which seizure activity spreads.

Corpus callosotomy may be used for severe atonic or tonic seizures (drop attacks), in children with a complex pattern of seizures such as the Lennox–Gastaut syndrome, in severe, uncontrolled generalized convulsions and in partial seizures with multiple seizure sources when the seizure spreads rapidly to the entire brain (becomes generalized).

A pioneering technique, *multiple subpial transection (MST)*, is used in crucial areas of the brain which control speech and movement. This involves very fine slicing of the cortex so as to stop epileptic activity moving across it, while leaving the essential nerve connections intact.

Techniques for the future focus on removing damaged tissue with minimal cutting through the skull and brain. Computer imaging techniques allow for greater precision and smaller incisions. *Stereotactic surgery* involves careful planning by computer beforehand, and an opening in the skull no bigger than the piece or pieces of tissue being removed. The latest addition to this type of surgery is the removal of scar tissue with a laser gamma knife, which avoids opening the skull at all. It has been used experimentally throughout much of the 1990s, but only very recently on patients with epilepsy. In 1997 a trial was carried out in France on a small group of patients who all had temporal lobe epilepsy, but for the time being it remains experimental rather than widely available for epilepsy.

■ VAGUS NERVE STIMULATION (VNS)

Still new, VNS has been arousing increasing interest, as well as a heated debate amongst the medical profession as to its usefulness – growing numbers of people have been trying it. It involves mild electrical stimulation of the vagus nerve, which carries information to the brain. Although it is not a cure for epilepsy, this treatment may halt seizures and improve the quality of life of some people. Recently approved in the US for adults and teenagers over 12 with hard-to-control seizures that begin in one part of the brain, it may also be successful with younger children.

A kind of pacemaker, a small device rather like a coin, is implanted in the chest under the collar bone in an operation under general anaesthetic lasting one to three hours. Wires lead from the generator to the vagus nerve, the largest nerve to leave the brain, which carries messages to and from it and controls heart rate and the digestive system.

Neurologists can set the implant to fire electrical signals to the brain for, say, about 30 seconds, every five minutes, 24 hours a day. The settings can be changed according to individual needs, and some people who feel a seizure coming on between programmed doses can also use a small magnet to make the device fire itself. In a very few people, the device may increase seizures, and if this happens it can be turned off using the magnet.

The electrical signals control seizures in some patients, although it is not yet known exactly how. It is thought that the nerve fibres in the vagus nerve are connected to areas of the brain believed to be involved in producing seizures. Stimulation of the vagus nerve may be able to intercept this abnormal brain activity. Some people using VNS may be able to reduce their medication after a while.

Case Study

Barbara, 11, was one of 80 patients with epilepsy to have a VNS implant done at King's College, London. The results are still being monitored, but her mother, Penny, says that her seizures have decreased noticeably. 'Previously she had so many a day you couldn't count them. It was as if someone were fiddling with a radio so that the sound was going on and off constantly and you had no real idea what the programme was about. She now has about 10–20 a day that we see. Her speech has also improved, and I'm sure the VNS has something to do with it.'

Some people may feel a tingling in the neck and become hoarse while the device is actually firing. Other side-effects reported by some include coughing, voice alteration, shortness of breath or a feeling of choking, throat pain, and ear or tooth pain. These sensations may become less noticeable over time. It can also be helpful to have the settings changed so that the stimulation is less long or strong. Other possible effects include skin irritation or infection at the implant side, problems with the device itself, inflammation and damage to the facial nerves or muscles. But VNS is still very new and only a few people have been treated by this method, so long-term side-effects have not yet been established.

The device is powered by a battery which lasts around three to five years. Estimates of the cost range from $8,000 to $15,000 in the USA (though it is sometimes available on the NHS in the UK). In the long term there will be compensating savings in things such as anti-epileptic drugs, routine hospital visits and emergency treatment after injury from seizures.

You can discuss the possibility of VNS with your own doctor and ask for a referral to a specialist, but bear in mind there is as yet no way of predicting who will respond to the treatment.

VNS research

According to the American Epilepsy Federation, in a recent study of 454 patients with poorly controlled seizures at 45 medical centres in the USA, Canada and Europe, most patients showed at least some improvement. Half the patients treated had at least a 20 per cent reduction in number of seizures per day. In about 25 per cent, the frequency of seizures decreased by more than 50 per cent. In about one in five, however, the seizures got worse.

According to the British Epilepsy Association, in the UK, where more than 100 people have had VNS, some studies suggest that around 15 per cent of patients stop having seizures at once, while most of the remaining patients will have a 50 per cent reduction in their seizure fequrency over the next 18 months, with continuing improvements. Seizures may also become less severe. A minority of patients will experience no improvement in their seizure pattern. Other studies, however, suggest that VNS may not be as successful as was initially hoped.

Chapter Four

Complementary Therapies

Case Study

'I'd certainly be interested in exploring natural therapies, but I don't know enough about it,' says Penny, mother of Barbara, 11. 'I do massage her back at night to get her to relax, and if she looks like she's going to have a seizure. I was also going to try reflexology, more as a relaxation again than as a cure, because she gets so agitated before a seizure, and if you can stop her panicking, you can sometimes stop the seizure.'

Interest in complementary therapies has been steadily gaining ground over the past few years as more and more people take responsibility for their own health – in the UK, an estimated 17 million people have consulted a natural therapist and recent surveys show consistent satisfaction levels of 60–80 per cent. There are several reasons why alternative medicine is popular.

- It gives people a sense of control.
- In particular, it empowers the patient by saying that the body has its own mechanisms of healing which it can use to get better. 'The natural healing force within each of us is the greatest force in getting well,' as Hippocrates said.
- It recognizes people's frustration with the limits of conventional medicine and the mechanistic, reductionist view of a person as a physical body made up of various pieces. Instead,

it presents a holistic view which acknowledges that a person is more than the sum of his physical parts.
- It goes well beyond health issues and encompasses philosophical, social, environmental and spiritual concerns.

The main fear among the conventional medical establishment is that this kind of philosophy might cause people to endanger their health by neglecting real health problems. This is a very valid concern in epilepsy, where suddenly stopping anti-epileptic drugs can be life-threatening. Certainly, people with epilepsy are strongly advised to maintain their conventional drug regimes strictly, to keep in regular contact with their usual epilepsy doctors, and not to make any changes without consulting them first. It is, however, increasingly recognized that complementary therapies have a part to play in improving health, and that conventional and complementary therapies do not have to be mutually exclusive but can and do work together very effectively.

One of the disadvantages of complementary or alternative medicine is that it is a blanket term so that a whole pot-pourri of remedies are grouped together under this one title, some of which are less well accredited than others. Indeed, natural remedies for epilepsy are an under-researched area, where the tendency is for individuals to branch out alone and try certain remedies in a rather hit-and-miss way (not like eczema, for example, which is known to respond well to many therapies such as traditional Chinese medicine). Many parents have thought of trying natural remedies for their child's epilepsy, but simply do not know where to start. Some of the therapies in this chapter have received attention and research from conventional medicinal practitioners; others have not, although some anecdotal evidence is positive. All are included, however, as alternatives to the mainstream practice of treating seizures with drugs.

To get the best out of natural remedies, follow these guidelines.

- It is vital to choose a practitioner with whom you feel at ease. Take your time, and ask other people – word of mouth remains the best recommendation. Staff in health-food shops are often knowledgeable.

- Give remedies a chance to work. Many natural therapies will make your child feel worse before he feels better – the so-called 'healing crisis' or 'aggravation reaction'. This means that symptoms get worse at first and, according to some practitioners, it is a sign that the treatment is working. However, if the deterioration is too severe, you should seek further advice.

- Above all, stay away from any therapist who suggests that your child gives up anti-epileptic medication, or that you cut all links with conventional medicine. Inform your doctor of what you are doing, and, if your child needs urgent medical help, contact the nearest hospital emergency department or your doctor.

DIETARY THERAPIES

The ketogenic diet

To quote the American neurologist John Freeman, of the Johns Hopkins Medical Institutions, Baltimore, one of the most favourable comments doctors made about the ketogenic diet in the past was 'Yuk!' Previously regarded as hopelessly unpalatable, it is a high-fat, low-carbohydrate diet which has to be started in hospital under the guidance of an experienced dietician and epilepsy team, and must then be monitored by a physician. Developed under the auspices of conventional medicine, it is not really a complementary therapy as it needs medical supervision, but it has fallen so far out of fashion that it more or less constitutes an alternative to mainstream drug practices, and so is included in this chapter.

When the ketogenic diet was first used, anti-epileptic medicine was not as developed as it is today, and, as soon as more effective drugs were evolved, it was on the whole swiftly and thankfully dropped. Not only was it unpalatable, it was – and is – also a great deal of trouble to follow. Since then, however, it has made something of a revival, especially in the USA.

The ketogenic diet begins with a day or so's fasting and then goes on to a food intake made up of 80–90 per cent fat, such as butter, cream, oils, eggs and fat meat, while cutting down strictly on carbohydrates such as bread, rice, pasta and sugar. Specifically designed for children with epilepsy, it originated in the 1920s after a New York paediatrician, Dr R M Wilder, observed that three patients who fasted with a faith healer temporarily stopped having seizures. It has been recognized for centuries that fasting may stop seizures, as it produces a condition called ketosis, when the body begins breaking down fat cells and produces acids called ketones, which are used for fuel and energy. In some people, especially children, this creates a metabolic state which prevents seizures. Like fasting, the high-fat intake creates ketosis as the body, deprived of carbohydrates (which would normally convert to glucose which would then be used for energy) is forced to use the ketones for fuel and energy.

It is not known exactly how the diet works but it is thought to affect the way the brain metabolizes ketones, which in turn affects seizure activity. Another theory is that the high fat levels help repair the myelin sheaths around the nerves of the brain. Myoclonic and atonic seizures respond best, and the diet is also used in the Lennox–Gastaut syndrome, but it can be used in all types of epilepsy.

Results are variable and it does not work for everyone. Improvements may be seen in the first weeks, but it is recommended that the diet is tried for one to three months before giving up as some children take longer to respond than others. It needs to be followed for at least two years, just as anti-epileptic medication does. Some parents have experienced good results from the diet, but others are less positive about it.

Case Studies

'She seemed much happier when taken off anti-epileptic drugs,' reports Debbie, mother of six-month-old Fay. 'She's started smiling again now and it's wonderful to see her lifting up her head again.'

Charlie, father of three-year-old Chrissie, agrees. 'Her speech went backwards at a rate of knots while on all the drugs, and she'd just come out with single words or baby words. Now she's talking in whole sentences. Physically she's caught up too, and is riding a tricycle with no problems.'

'You have to be pretty desperate to try it,' says Nancy, mother of six-year-old Tyson. 'It's very hard work and only controls our son's seizures by day – he takes a cocktail of drugs and still has multiple seizures at night.'

Five-year-old Lily's diet resulted in failure. 'We tried the keto diet for about six weeks,' says her mother, Sue. But at the time Lily didn't like cream and we couldn't get any creamy, milky drinks down her. In fact we found the rest of the diet easy enough to arrange with the help of a dietician, but it didn't work. Lily was hungry and grumpy all the time, and above all, it had no effect – we got her ketones going quite well, but her seizures remained the same.'

You should consider the following points when deciding whether to try the ketogenic diet with your child.

- It is a stringent diet, and every bit of food needs to be carefully weighed and measured.
- Even tiny intakes of extra carbohydrate, such as a mouthful of biscuit, can break the diet and result in a seizure, so you may have to allow for some upset if mistakes are made or your child cheats.

- The diet lacks essential nutrients such as vitamins B and C and calcium, which must be given as sugar-free supplements.
- Toothpaste, vitamins and medicines may have enough sugar in them to break the diet and need careful monitoring with your doctor.
- The diet can be modified for children who are allergic to or intolerant of milk and milk products, but this may take more planning.
- The diet has side-effects, sometimes severe, including higher cholesterol levels (including very high levels (hyper-cholesterolemia), the long-term effects of which on children are not yet known), constipation, kidney stones, vomiting, dehydration, anaemia, loss of minerals in the bones, recurrent infections and lethargy.
- Your child's growth may slow down slightly as he gains little weight on a properly calculated diet. However, after two years, children usually catch up rapidly.
- It needs a doctor experienced in the diet to help you through it – this is emphatically not something to try on your own as a self-help remedy. For how to get hold of more information on the ketogenic diet, ask your family doctor or epilepsy specialist, or see the 'Further Reading' and 'Useful Addresses' sections at the end of this book.

Keto research
According to the Epilepsy Federation of America, research shows that about a third of children on the ketogenic diet have very good or complete seizure control, a third have improved seizure control, while the last third do not benefit from the diet or find the side-effects too much and do not stay on the diet very long.

In one study of 68 children at the Johns Hopkins Hospital, Baltimore, 59 per cent remained on the diet for more than a year and 32 per cent of all the children were seizure-free. The diet was discontinued in 41 per cent of patients because of poor seizure control or poor tolerance. Children under ten tended to achieve better seizure control than those over ten, but both groups had substantial improvement with a majority reporting more than a 50 per cent reduction in seizure frequency.

In a similar study involving 63 children from the University of Utah, more than a third had their seizures reduced by 75 per cent or more. And researchers at Stanford University found that two-thirds of the children they studied had their seizures reduced by more than half, while 16 per cent were able to stop taking anti-epileptic medication.

The Ketogenic diet: sample foods
The following list gives a general idea of the type of foods your child might expect to eat on the ketogenic diet. It is not intended to be followed, and you should not try to start your child on this kind of diet without medical supervision. As every child's epilepsy is different, food intake needs to be individually prescribed to the last gram.

Breakfast: egg scrambled with butter; bacon; sausage; fruit; popcorn and butter
Lunch (main meal): steak; lettuce with mayonnaise dressing; raw vegetable salad (eg broccoli) with mayonnaise dressing; minced lamb burger with vegetables browned with crushed garlic and parmesan cheese; maize tacos with minced beef, sour cream, lettuce strips and melted cheese; aubergine stewed with cream and cheese
Dinner (light meal): eggs baked in spinach with cream and cheese; pink/red salmon with fresh spinach leaves or iceberg lettuce and olive oil; asparagus and cottage cheese salad with garlic mayonnaise; pancakes stuffed with tofu, ketchup and grated cheese; chicken strips or vegetable pieces in mayonnaise dip; chunks of banana or melon dipped in whipped cream; crackers with butter and peanut butter
To drink: diluted cream; milkshake; ice cream soda (made with natural ingredients and no sugar)

An Indian study suggests the following diet (for one day): 6oz butter or ghee, or clarified butter; two eggs; two pieces bread or chapati; 10oz whole milk; 2oz meat or dal-bean sauce; 8oz mixed vegetables; and one orange.

Work on the ketogenic diet at Booth Hall Children's Hospital, Manchester, suggests that 50–70 per cent of the calories be given as medium-chain triglycerides (MCT), a type of oil which can be used for frying or grilling, in baked foods, and as a drink mixed with gelatin and milk. However, other researchers suggest that the older-style, heavy-fat diet is more effective than one containing MCT oil.

Boosting nutrients

Nutritional therapists have linked various vitamin and mineral deficiencies with epilepsy, either because an individual's diet is deficient, or because he suffers from malabsorption syndrome, when the body cannot use the nutrients (eg coeliac disease, *see* pages 88–9). It seems that in some cases shortages of nutrients are what tip the balance in children with epileptic brain activity and result in an actual seizure.

One of the most important of these is *calcium deficiency (hypocalcaemia)* which, though comparatively rare, has been identified as a metabolic disorder especially in newborn babies. In particular, early feeding with cows' milk may contribute to low calcium levels, as this is very high in phosphates, which in fact cause the body to excrete calcium. (In older children, fizzy drinks are also high in phosphorus and can pose a real threat to calcium levels.) Calcium is vital to normal brain functioning, and in some children too much calcium may be lost through the urine as a result of kidney disease. So if you do suspect low calcium as a cause of seizures, you should seek the advice of your conventional practitioner, as the root cause may need medical investigation. Otherwise, the best sources of calcium are milk and dairy products, although if your child cannot tolerate milk, other good sources include bony fish (eg sardines), seeds, nuts (especially almonds), dried figs, bread and dark leafy green vegetables.

Lack of magnesium, which interacts with calcium, can also contribute to seizures. Magnesium can also occasionally be lost in the urine because of kidney inflammation (nephritis). Some studies have found that extra magnesium stops seizures to the point where drugs can be discontinued. Some people have bene- fited from combining supplements of vitamin B6 and magnesium. Magnesium is found in wholemeal flour, millet, figs, meat, fish, nuts and pulses.

Vitamin B6 (pyridoxine deficiency) is another recognized cause of seizures in newborn babies, and a hospital paediatrician may suggest extra doses of this vitamin if a baby is convulsing. Lesser symptoms of B6 deficiency or dependency, other than seizures, include irritability, sensitivity to noise and abnormal EEGs. This is due to a rare metabolic condition in which the baby's body chemistry needs unusually large doses of vitamin B6. Your paedi- atrician may occasionally suggest extra vitamin B6 for an older child, too, although some people have found that this has little effect. Vitamin B6 is also recognized as being helpful for stress and emotional swings, so it may well be worth making sure that your child's diet includes adequate amounts of this vitamin. Good sources of vitamin B6 include meat, whole grains and pulses. A vitamin B complex supplement could also help, to make sure that your child's intake of all the B vitamins (which are necessary to maintain the central nervous system) remains balanced – increasing your intake of vitamin B6 means an increased need for other B vitamins, such as B2, and pantothenic acid. Do discuss supplementation with your doctor.

Other vitamin shortages may include: *folic acid* (made worse by some anti-epileptic drugs, although it is inadvisable to sup- plement this without guidance as large doses of folic acid have been known to make epilepsy worse); *vitamin D* (important both in its own right and as helping the absorption of calcium), which is found in most oily fish and some animal products, especially in cheese and fortified milks; and *vitamin E*, important for oxygen flow round the body.

Mineral deficiencies associated with epilepsy include *iron deficiency (anaemia)*, which may be a problem if your child suffers frequent digestive troubles or a teenage girl has heavy periods.

Anaemia is also recognized as a common problem in toddlers. Good sources of iron include red meat, eggs, sardines, dried fruit such as apricots, and nuts such as almonds.

Zinc is important for brain functioning and helps raise levels of taurine in the brain (*see* below). It works best in combination with manganese. Zinc is found in meat and offal, wheatgerm, nuts, crab, oysters and lentils.

Some research also suggests a link between congenital seizures and deficiency of *manganese* in the expectant mother's diet. Good sources of manganese include watercress, okra, oats, rice, wholemeal bread, wheatgerm, buckwheat, lima beans, nuts, cockles, sardines, blackberries, figs and pineapple.

Finally, *taurine* is an amino acid that helps inhibit neuronal activity, and some people with epilepsy have found that taking extra doses helps control their seizures. *Di-methyl glycine (DMG)* is another amino acid which helps oxygen move round the system and has been shown to bring people out of a seizure.

Diet – why you need expert advice

Nutrient deficiency can be due to a wide range of causes, including stress and pollution, so you should get expert advice from your usual doctor or from an experienced, qualified nutritional therapist.

Correcting deficiencies should be part of an overall nutrition programme. It certainly will not hurt if you improve your family's diet following the guidelines in chapter 2, but your child may also benefit from a regime which is individually prescribed by a therapist who understands epilepsy and knows which drugs he is on.

Some anti-epileptic drugs deplete nutrients and your child's doctor may routinely prescribe supplements; otherwise, check with a qualified practitioner before rushing out to buy extra vitamins and minerals. Supplementation really needs expert guidance to avoid further imbalance.

▦ Detoxification

A build-up of various toxins, such as chemicals used in foods, pesticides and pollution, has been associated with epilepsy. Obviously it helps to buy organic food but this may be difficult, and it is likewise often impossible to avoid pollution, but there are still steps you can take to detoxify your child's system. A water filter from a health food shop will remove chemicals from your drinking water as well as metals such as aluminium and copper – heavy-metal toxicity has in particular been associated with epilepsy. You can also consult a nutritional therapist, who may be able to prescribe special supplements for individual problems. For example, heavy-metal toxicity can be dealt with by chelation therapy, which detoxifies the body using certain vitamins and minerals which wash the heavy metals out of the system.

See if you can get your child to eat more fresh fruit and vegetables – perhaps juiced with a juice extractor, in soups or in purees such as aubergine or guacamole (avocado). The vitamin C they contain is a good detoxicant. Garlic is also often recommended for helping the body work more efficiently, and for helping elimination.

Case Study

The parents of Robert, aged five, began to suspect that pesticides played a part in his epilepsy after a holiday abroad when they stayed with friends on a banana plantation, and Robert twice had seizures soon after the trees were sprayed. When they got home, they took action. They peeled all fruit and vegetables, bought organic food wherever possible, and installed a domestic reverse-osmosis system for drinking water. They also discovered that Robert seemed to be allergic to a certain brand of deodorant, and to the fabric softener his mother used when washing clothes. His seizures were much reduced, although at seven he continues to take medication. His parents are delighted that his condition is now almost under control, whereas previously he was still having frequent seizures despite taking medication.

Food allergy and intolerance

While many conventional doctors will tell you that genuine food allergy is much more rare than people think, it is acknowledged that intolerances to food and environmental substances are rising rapidly, and many parents of children with epilepsy believe that their children's seizures take place in reaction to certain foods. At Great Ormond Street Hospital for Sick Children in London, a study done on children with migraine and epilepsy found that once allergies and intolerances had been identified and the culprit foods removed, both migraine and epilepsy disappeared in 78 out of 88 children.

One clue to whether your child suffers from allergies or intolerances may be if he also suffers from other allergy- or intolerance-related illnesses such as hayfever and eczema. Another is that, after eating something to which he is allergic or intolerant, his pulse may start racing – although obviously to be sure you should have his nutritional status analysed by an expert.

Suspect an allergy or intolerance to wheat and other gluten-containing foods first (rye, barley, oats, buckwheat). Foods which contain wheat are legion, and you may need to read the ingredient lists on prepared foods (including vitamin and mineral supplements) to avoid it completely. An extreme form of wheat allergy is coeliac disease, in which the body is prevented from absorbing nutrients (malabsorption syndrome) by persistent diarrhoea, vomiting and poor appetite. It is thought to be due to an inability to digest wheat gluten, which contains an intestinal irritant, gliadin. Coeliac disease may put people at greater risk of seizures in particular because it washes nutrients such as iron and calcium through the system, so creating deficiencies which predispose to seizures.

Coeliac disease and epilepsy research
Several medical studies have linked coeliac disease (CD) with epilepsy. In a study of 783 patients with seizures by the Institute of Clinical Pediatrics at the University of Siena, Italy, symptoms of CD were found in some patients, which had been previously overlooked. And, interestingly given the link with calcium deficiency mentioned above, a study of CD and hypocalcaemia at the Department of Neurology at Hadassah University Hospital, Jerusalem, concluded that malabsorption put patients at increased risk of seizures, and recommended that even a mild degree of hypocalcaemia should be corrected as soon as possible.

Other common allergens include milk and dairy products, sugar, eggs, peanuts, citrus fruits, strawberries, shellfish, food additives and preservatives and tap water. The artificial sweetener aspartame has been linked to seizures by research at Arizona State University.

Try improving the family's general diet, as sometimes allergic-type symptoms can occur if a child is lacking nutrients. A nutritional therapist may also suggest an elimination diet to try to find the food which is causing the problem. An elimination diet will usually start by excluding all foods except those known to cause very few allergies, such as lamb, rabbit and spinach. After a few days, more foods are reintroduced to see if there is a reaction (sometimes a reaction can take place as much as 18–24 hours after eating). You could also try a hypo-allergenic diet, which excludes the main allergens (*see* below).

The hypo-allergenic diet
The Society for the Promotion of Nutritional Therapy in the UK suggests that the following hypo-allergenic diet be followed for about two weeks. It avoids common potential allergens, although there may be withdrawal symptoms, such as headaches or nausea, for a few days. You could then try reintroducing foods to see if there is a reaction.

Eat freely:

- fresh or frozen fruit and vegetables
- fresh or frozen fish
- nuts and seeds
- beans and pulses such as lentils, chickpeas, kidney beans (check that tinned varieties do not contain sugar)
- soya products such as tofu and soya milk (but avoid soy sauce as it contains wheat)
- cold-pressed unrefined oils such as sunflower, sesame and extra virgin olive oil
- non-gluten grains such as brown rice, millet and buckwheat
- herbal teas
- natural sweeteners such as small amounts of honey and maple syrup

Avoid:

- milk and dairy products such as butter, cheese and yoghurt
- wheat and other sources of gluten – oats, bread, pastry, pasta, cakes, ready-made sauce mixes etc.
- animal protein – red or white meat and eggs
- stimulants – sugar, tea, coffee and alcohol
- sweets and chocolates
- convenience foods
- yeast (as in yeast extract)

Case Study

Gail was six when she drank some lemonade at a birthday party, vomited it straight up again, and had one of her tonic–clonic seizures. Her parents blamed overexcitement initially, but when she did the same again after drinking another soft drink, they decided to investigate further. They took her to a nutritional therapist who said she was allergic to sugar and artificial sweeteners, as well as to dairy products. He also recommended that they cut out refined foods and foods containing additives as far as possible (refined flour, bought biscuits, cakes etc.). These measures helped reduce seizures immediately, although they were not brought under complete control until Gail had epilepsy surgery (a callosotomy) a year later.

BODY THERAPIES

Alexander technique

The Alexander technique aims to teach the body how to hold itself and move correctly. Its founder, F Matthias Alexander, an actor working in the 1920s, believed that many of us pick up bad habits of posture and movement which then affect our health, mood and general wellbeing. The technique aims to realign the head so that it sits correctly in line with the spine.

It has been recommended for people with epilepsy because in a tonic–clonic seizure the musculo-skeletal framework may be thrust out of alignment by the violent physical activity involved. As well as helping realign the whole framework, the technique may help your child conserve energy and move less tensely. It may also help him breathe in a more relaxed way; this can be an important factor in controlling seizures which have a slow onset with a recognizable warning.

Yoga

Yoga may appeal particularly to children, as many of the body postures or *asanas* are based on animals – the cat, the cobra, the lion and the rabbit, to name but a few, which children often enjoy imitating, complete with relevant sound effects! Yoga is a Sanskrit term deriving from *yuj*, which means to harness horses to a chariot – perhaps a relevant metaphor if you view a seizure as uncontrolled energy which carries the victim out of control.

Yoga forms a kind of bridge between body and mind, and it has many benefits for children. It improves suppleness, muscle tone, strength and poise, and gives extra bodily confidence and awareness, so making for a more positive self-image – which is vital, given epilepsy's potential for decimating self-esteem. It can teach children to recognize stress, and what it feels like to be totally relaxed – a knowledge which many people do not attain, even in adulthood, and which is particularly relevant in view of the link between stress and epilepsy. The breathing exercises may be of special importance as some children can have seizures through hyperventilating, not to mention the fact that poor breathing is in itself a major cause of stress and less-than-perfect health.

On the mental and emotional level, yoga is gentle and not competitive. It gives children a chance to express their feelings without words, and teaches them that their bodies can be channels of creativity as well as of epileptic attacks. Children with a short attention span and frequent mood changes (which applies to all children but may have added relevance for those with epilepsy) may also find the practice of yoga postures helps improve their concentration. And the practice of yoga teaches children what it is like to care for themselves and take more responsibility for their bodies, which can have lifelong value in epilepsy.

If you decide to start doing yoga with your child, follow these guidelines.

- Take the poses slowly and smoothly; never rush them.
- Start with warm-up exercises and wind down with a short relaxation time.
- Make sure your child's stomach is fairly empty – do the exercises before breakfast, one hour after a light meal or two hours after a main meal.
- Make a game of the poses or keep session times short – just a few minutes – if your child looks as though he is becoming bored.
- If you are enrolling your child in a class, make sure the yoga teacher knows he has epilepsy.

If you are not sure whether yoga would suit your child, consult your doctor.

Cranial osteopathy and chiropractic

Cranial osteopathy is a form of very light head massage, which can help realign any bones which have been displaced by a difficult birth or other trauma. Because epilepsy has so many different root causes, cranial osteopathy cannot be prescribed as a blanket cure – or even as a cure at all. However, it may help improve your child's overall condition and so improve the epilepsy indirectly, especially in cases of micro-scarring after a head injury or traumatic birth which has stopped just short of causing brain damage.

Cranial osteopathy may help stabilize tiny movements of the brain, which may improve some epilepsy as well as contributing to general wellbeing. The brain has different rhythms and blood flows of its own, and osteopaths may also treat tiny aberrations of independent movements made by the brain within its fluid. By ensuring that the central nervous system is working as freely as possible, this helps the body's own self-healing mechanisms work better, too.

Osteopathy may benefit your child in different ways – for example, it has helped some babies with colic, and it may also help with sleeping problems, as cranial strain may disrupt parts of the brain which govern sleep.

Chiropractic can be described as a variant of osteopathy, and some people have found it even gentler. It works on the belief that aligning the spine can help lessen the strain on the nervous system.

Neither osteopathy nor chiropractic works for everyone – some people have reported that these methods seem to have triggered seizures. Your choice of practitioner may also be important – find someone who favours a very gentle, 'laying on of hands' type of technique.

▓ Herbal remedies

Some therapists have also used herbal medicine with success, perhaps combining it with other remedies such as homoeopathy (*see* pages 100–102). A herbalist will prescribe an individual mix of remedies for your child, which will take into account his overall health and any other existing conditions – in fact, like many other complementary remedies, it aims to treat the whole person and so improve general health. In addition, some therapists will assume something of a counselling role, and will aim to deal with emotional stresses and strains as part of the treatment.

Herbs, though natural, can be powerful, and should be treated with respect. In fact, much of today's work by pharmaceutical companies is based on traditional herbal remedies, and up to 70 per cent of conventional drugs in use today have their origins in plants. Do not buy over-the-counter remedies, and do check a herbalist's qualifications.

Herbs said to be good for epilepsy include blue vervain, hyssop, lobelia and skullcap.

▓ Naturopathy

Naturopathy is a truly holistic approach which involves treating a person with a mixture of different therapies. In epilepsy, a naturopath might look for nutritional imbalances and food allergies and intolerances, as well as considering psychological factors and exercises. Some naturopaths are qualified in other disciplines such as osteopathy and homoeopathy, and many make use also of hydrotherapy, which ranges from salt baths to bathing in warm thermal springs. Detoxification may also play an important part.

▨ BEHAVIOUR TRAINING THERAPIES

Many of the most successful 'alternative' remedies for epilepsy are behaviour training methods which involve quite a lot of work and willingness on the part of your child. Most of the work and studies in this area have been done on adults, but they can also be used by children too, and there is certainly no harm in asking your doctor or alternative practitioner if you feel your child might benefit. The idea behind them is that people can change the behaviour which leads up to a seizure – sometimes on quite a deep level, as efforts of concentration may actually change brainwave patterns. Some children use their own learned behaviour methods, such as running around or holding a comforter, to stop a seizure. Older children may read, or lie down and concentrate on something specific to maintain consciousness.

▨ Biofeedback

Biofeedback acts on the principle that our thoughts can control our bodies – even unconscious processes such as the brain's electrical activity. By using various instruments to measure how relaxed your child is, it can increase his awareness of his body and the physical signs of stress. For example, the skin becomes colder if one is stressed, because blood is directed to the heart, lungs and muscles, ready for 'fight or flight'. Biofeedback can measure temperature (thermal biofeedback) or muscle tension (electromyograph biofeedback). The instruments 'feed back' the information the body is giving out, convert it into a readable signal, and may be programmed to make a sound or display a light once a certain level of relaxation is achieved. Children may find this kind of biofeedback useful if they have seizures.

Biofeedback for epilepsy uses EEG to measure brain activity, which may then be shown as a computer image; your child has the power to change this using mental techniques which also control brain activity. Around a third of people with epilepsy can sometimes stop seizures this way, according to Peter Fenwick, consultant at London's Maudsley Hospital Institute of Psychiatry, who has done a lot of research into epilepsy and biofeedback. The technique has also been the subject of much research by Professor Nils Birbaumer of the Institute of Medical Psychology and Behavioural Neurobiology at the University of Tübingen, Germany. He and his team found that people were able to reduce the frequency and strength of seizures significantly after 20 sessions of biofeedback training.

Biofeedback works best with people who experience partial seizures or secondary generalized seizures, which begin with some kind of warning or aura, so that they have time to take action. This means that your child needs to be aware of (or to be taught how to recognize) the events and feelings which lead up to a seizure, which means that biofeedback needs to be accompanied by other psychological work and general epilepsy management – tools which can be useful generally in helping him exercise more control over his epilepsy, especially when used along with other methods such as diet and dealing with stress. In children where epilepsy is part of a range of disorders, it is also thought that other problems may respond to EEG training, such as mood or sleep disorders, or attention deficit problems.

Aromatherapy

Aromatherapy can be used slightly differently for epilepsy than normal, as it includes psychological components as well as being physically relaxing. Certain aromatherapy oils such as ylang ylang, lavender and camomile are usually viewed as relaxing, and used in conjunction with a soothing massage may be enough to ward off a seizure; like adults, some children have to be taught what it feels like to be truly relaxed. In addition, research work at Birmingham University has focused on creating a memory link between the smell of the oil and the state of relaxation, so that merely smelling the oil at a later date will evoke sensations of being relaxed. Patients at Birmingham University's Seizure Clinic also learned to use hypnosis or visualization techniques which reminded them of the relaxing 'smell memory' of the oil, and the relaxed state it evoked.

The smell of the oils works on the olfactory (smell) centres in the temporal lobes of the brain, which in turn affect the brain's limbic area, which is involved in the senses, mood control, instinctive behaviour and emotions. Of the original ten patients who were followed up for more than two years, six became seizure-free and three were able to withdraw from medication; later studies show similar encouraging results.

This is obviously a specialized area which demands commitment and psychological work from the patient, who may have to practise the techniques regularly to gain lasting advantage. However, there is no reason why your child should not benefit from the relaxing effects of aromatherapy massage – other research has found that a 20-minute back massage of various oils including melissa led to a reduction in seizures. But some aromatherapy oils are thought to stimulate the brain and seizure activity and should be avoided by people with epilepsy – they include hyssop, rosemary, sweet fennel and sage. An aromatherapist should always know about your child's epilepsy.

ENERGY THERAPIES

Energy therapies aim to rebalance, unblock or stimulate the flow of energy or the life force, which they believe has become unbalanced or blocked in illness. This life force has many different names in different cultures – in traditional Chinese medicine it is called qi, in India, prana. It has also been called od, odic force, orgone and bioplasma. Energy therapists believe that when the life force is at a high level, and flowing freely, people are less likely to become ill. The life force is believed to animate the body and to be the primary energy of our emotions, thoughts and spiritual life.

▦ Traditional Chinese medicine (TCM)

The Chinese place great importance on qi and believe that there are many different kinds – the *Yellow Emperor's Classic of Internal Medicine*, which is over 4,000 years old, lists 32 different kinds. Together with the *xue*, or blood, TCM practioners believe that qi must flow freely along the body's meridians or channels, and that a blockage or an imblance in qi components (yin and yang) can cause illness. For example, lack of rest and proper nutrition can weaken one's qi and so affect the emotional state, which in turn may affect seizure control in some people. Again, stress can adversely affect the emotions, cause qi to stagnate in the body and result in various physical complaints.

Chinese medicine, which requires at least five years' training, has a history of working with Western medicine since the latter's introduction into China in the 1840s. Many Chinese practitioners practise both kinds, and a reputable practitioner should be more than happy to work alongside family or hospital doctors.

TCM looks at the body as a whole, so a Chinese doctor will take a detailed medical history and give your child a thorough physical inspection which includes looking at the tongue (a traditional diagnostic tool in Chinese medicine), listening to his voice, noting any body odour and taking both wrist pulses to check various points which are believed to give information about the heart, liver, etc. Herbs, which are often imported directly from China, are used, and may include flowers, leaves, stalks, seeds and roots. A prescription may consist of as many as a dozen of these working in synergy. As Chinese herbal medicine has existed for many thousands of years, practitioners say that the understanding of their action and how to avoid side-effects has been passed on over countless generations, making this kind of therapy an extremely safe one. You must, however, consult a reputable practitioner and avoid self-prescribing.

According to TCM, epilepsy is diagnosed as phlegm or dampness caused by a blocked heart meridian. Generally, a TCM doctor will treat epilepsy with Chinese herbs which aim to restore balance within the body, such as sweet flag root, Chinese senegar root, bamboo shavings or bamboo juice. The aim is to treat the heart, the spleen and sometimes the liver. A strict diet may also be prescribed, for example excluding sugar, fried foods, most dairy products and alcohol.

Practitioners say that, while epilepsy is difficult to cure, TCM may help reduce the number of attacks, and in some cases stop them. With TCM, your child may also be able to reduce the dosage of prescribed drugs, although reputable doctors will encourage you to continue with at least a small dose of anti-epileptic drugs, as epilepsy cannot be controlled with TCM treatment alone. There is no reliable scientific research to show that TCM helps reduce the need for drugs, so it is very important that you double check with your doctor before attempting any drug reduction.

Acupuncture

Acupuncture may be used after or together with herbal remedies in TCM, and studies at the Shanghai College of Traditional Chinese Medicine and the Xiamen Hospital of Traditional Chinese Medicine have investigated its use in epilepsy. It is not clear exactly how acupuncture may be beneficial in cases of epilepsy, but it has been found to be an effective relaxation therapy, as it helps the body release endorphins (painkilling hormones) and so may help children who tend to have more seizures when stressed and anxious. It has also been suggested that acupuncture works on the brain's limbic centre, which is connected with moods and behaviour, and is often implicated in epilepsy.

The needles are inserted at key points along the body to access the 12 channels (meridians) where qi flows through the body. The meridians are said to influence different organs and body systems.

Acupuncture should be approached with care and is certainly not for everyone, as there are reports of it actually causing seizures, sometimes as the needles go in. Instead of needles, practitioners may use variants of acupuncture, such as the massage of acupuncture points (acupressure), which children are likely to prefer to the traditional needle technique.

Shiatsu, which is often linked with acupuncture, also involves the massage of the key points of the body in order to stimulate the qi. Some parents familiar with the technique have tried it as a relaxing massage for their children, and it may work well in combination with other remedies such as diet.

Case Study

Frances took her eight-year-old son Paul to a Chinese practitioner for a combination of hay fever and epilepsy. 'I came home with bags and bags of weird-looking (and smelling!) herbs – one lot I actually called my neighbour in to look at as I'm convinced it was bits of dried locusts. Many of the herbs had to be boiled for quite a while – once I forgot a saucepan of them for an hour and came back to find the kitchen full of black smoke!' In spite of such mishaps, however, Paul's seizures decreased. The TCM doctor also prescribed a strict diet – no chocolate, no sweets, no milk or dairy products, and no refined or convenience foods. Paul did not think much of this but managed to stick to it (with the odd lapse). When the time came to return to the hospital, he was able to take a minimal amount of medication instead of the heavier dose the consultant originally planned to prescribe, and Frances hopes that in time Paul may even be able to give up drugs completely.

Homoeopathy

Homoeopaths aim to bring a person's system into balance, and use a wide range of remedies made up of substances such as plants, minerals and metals. It has achieved some success with some children with epilepsy, although results are variable. Remedies are individually prescribed, so no blanket statement can be made about which remedy suits which child, but treatments which have been used to treat epilepsy include argentum nitricum, caulophyllum, causticum, cicuta, cocculus, crotalus, cuprum, glonomium, ignatia, nux vomica, plumbum and pulsatilla.

Homoeopaths sometimes also make use of flower remedies, minute extracts of flower essences which many believe have a powerful effect on the body's energy system. The best known of these are the Bach flower remedies, but other types, such as the Californian and Bush remedies, have also become popular.

Case Studies
Elizabeth was 14, and when she started menstruating she went through a bad few days of hyperventilating and feeling panicky. She also suffered from asthma which became worse around this time. She had a seizure with almost every period. She was given cuprum to take in the week before her period, and the seizures stopped.

Before starting Natalie on a course of drugs, her mother Jocelyn asked the family doctor for three months' grace while she had a look at alternative remedies. He agreed with reluctance, and warned her that there was a risk that untreated epilepsy would only get worse. Jocelyn found a homoeopath who suggested two flower remedies and a homoeopathic remedy. He took a holistic approach and felt, as did Jocelyn, that Natalie's problems were being made worse by family stresses, including her father's very negative attitude to her recently diagnosed epilepsy. He seemed to be unable to accept that she was no longer his 'perfect' little girl, and ignored or shouted at her.

Under the homoeopathic treatment, Natalie's tonic–clonic seizures dropped in frequency to about one every two months, and she now only has the occasional absence. Her relationship with her father also improved as he became interested in the homoeopathic treatment and felt that by supporting it he was doing something for her epilepsy, whereas previously he had felt helpless with the hospital doctors.

Reflexology

Reflexology, which was in use in ancient China, India and Egypt, has been recommended as a complementary therapy for people with epilepsy. Therapists believe that the flow of qi can be stimulated, and health improved, by finger and thumb massage of the feet, as parts of the foot are believed to correspond to parts of the body. While reflexology can be relaxing, overstimulation can trigger seizures in some people, and reflexologists are usually taught to treat people with epilepsy cautiously and gently.

Healing

Case Study
Meena, 16, had six sessions with a healer-therapist, who worked on her general mental, emotional and spiritual health, in particular the depression around seizures which had been afflicting her for a couple of years. With this treatment, she was able to achieve much better emotional balance, which helped both her depression and her seizure control, although she says the effects were subtle, not dramatic, and took a while to make themselves felt – in fact, it took her four or five weeks after the first two sessions to realize that she was feeling better.

Healing is not about curing epilepsy, or indeed about miraculous cures of any condition. It deals more with the transfer of energy from healer to patient, a transaction which may involve psychologically shedding one's burdens and feeling more spiritually balanced. Healers work in different ways – laying on of hands, distance healing and deep psychological work to identify any negativity which could be blocking health and happiness.

How does healing work? The philosophy behind much healing

has its roots in ancient Taoist, Buddhist and Hindu philosophies, which view matter and energy as inextricably interwoven – indeed, modern quantum physics also holds that matter and energy are interchangeable. Matter exists in a dynamic energy field and cannot be separated from its activity. This means that explanations have to go beyond the cause-and-effect approach of modern science, and take on more fluid, dynamic concepts such as process and transformation. Five factors are said to play a part in the healing process:

1 **High levels of qi.** Qi levels may vary according to area. For example, some mountains or springs (such as the springs at Lourdes) are believed to have a higher life force than usual; some rooms in the house may also have more potent energy.
2 **The patient's attitude.** Fear, distrust and guilt may be barriers to healing – some healers say children are easier to heal because of their trusting attitude. However, it may not be necessary to believe in the healing to benefit from it.
3 **Relaxation.** Both healer and patient should be able to relax.
4 **Love.** The healer must be filled with love and compassion for the patient, and a desire to see him get well. These feelings do not have to be personal.
5 **Asking a higher power to help.** Healers ask for help from a universal God or power, however that is interpreted, and thank this power for help received.

Healers may work in an altered state of consciousness, a 'clair-voyant reality' which takes into account people's psychic as well as their physical state. Innate intuition, meditation and practice may help healers achieve this state, although it remains unpredictable, as do the results, which sceptics believe are due to short-term psychological effects. However, it is possible that actively participating in the treatment may help some children, who may feel they are taking more responsibility for their own health by joining in a healing session. It is also possible that the special attention is beneficial to some children! In the UK, healers work according to a code which forbids them to promise miracle cures, and may be members of the National Federation of Spiritual Healers.

There are many different kinds of healing. *Therapeutic touch* is laying on of hands or light massage, which is believed to transmit the universal life force or qi. One of the women who developed it, Dora van Gelder Kunz, a meditation teacher, saw the healing process as taking part in a universe where all things are interconnected, and both healer and patient as expressions of a 'unified therapeutic interaction'. This thinking still underlies much of today's healing work.

The therapist scans the patient's body with his hands, looking for imbalances in the energy flow which may feel uneven, cold or bare, depending on the individual healer's perception. He then uses light hand movements to release and restore any blocked or lacking energy. Many people find this very relaxing and soothing, which can in itself be enough to help lessen seizures.

Therapeutic touch has received a lot of interest from the nursing profession, especially in the USA, where the American Holistic Nurses Association has been set up, and Canada, where it has been incorporated into the 1990 Standard of Practice of the College of Nurses in Ontario.

Reiki, the Usui system of natural healing, is a technique which aims to connect with the life force or universal energy to improve health and enhance the quality of life. Reiki healers believe the ability to use Reiki is not taught in the usual sense, but is transferred to the student during four initiation ceremonies with a Reiki master.

Reiki is believed to be spiritually guided, and works to restore harmony. Treatment may vary, but it usually involves simply placing the hands on another person and keeping them still for several minutes, during which time many beneficial effects can become apparent. (Reiki initiates can also try this healing process on themselves which means there is no reason why people with epilepsy should not aim to 'train' as Reiki masters themselves.) Reiki, which aims to work on the cause of a problem rather than its symptoms, treats the whole person, including body, emotions, mind and spirit, though what happens in each treatment varies according to individual needs and readiness to change. People treated often describe deep relaxation and feelings of peace, security and wellbeing. However, people who give Reiki do not see themselves as healing the other person, as the Reiki view is that a person can only heal himself. Instead, they see their role as helping the student connect with healing energies, and creating a safe environment in which this kind of self-healing may take place. No particular beliefs are needed in order to practise or receive Reiki.

SHEN therapy was developed in California in the 1990s by Richard Pavek, who claims to have cured a person of epilepsy. SHEN therapy itself, however, makes no specific claims, which its practitioners feel would be wrong and against the spirit of the treatment.

The therapy seems to aim to release blocked energy, which therapists do by a mixture of laying on of hands and massage. Normally, according to SHEN therapists, energy circulates and clears via a number of exits in the body, such as the solar plexus, heart and throat. Once these exits become blocked, ill health can be the result.

According to some SHEN therapists, as the energy clears, emotional conflicts, wounds or deep fears, which have been long held in the body's memory and which some therapists believe are manifested as convulsions, may also be released. In this psychological release of unresolved emotional trauma, SHEN resembles gestalt therapy, though SHEN involves no words, in order to respect individual liberty. While it aims to create a safe environment in which this kind of release may take place, the release mechanism does appear from anecdotal reports to be quite a powerful experience, so it may be doubly important to make sure you choose a practitioner with whom you feel at ease.

Healing and the aura

Some healers diagnose after seeing disturbances in the body's energy field or aura (not the aura or warning which comes before some epileptic seizures). The aura is believed to be a vibrating energy form thrown out several feet around the body. Healers who believe there is no mind/body divide perceive the aura as another manifestation of the same energy which makes up the body. Some psychically gifted healers can see specific colours in the aura, and can 'scan' the area with their psychic or spiritual eyes and detect disturbances in it which may reflect physical weaknesses or illnesses. Many alternative healers believe that by healing the aura, the body is also healed. They also believe that this should not be at the expense of basic, sensible bodily care, and that a holistic approach, with a healthy diet and lifestyle and as little negativity as possible, is best for rebalancing energies and maintaining overall health.

Chapter Five

As They Grow

Case Studies

'Barbara is very open about her epilepsy,' says Penny, her mother. ' "I have epilepsy" is almost the first thing she says when opening the door to someone. We have to try to teach her – very tactfully! – that all the world may not be a friend.'

Christopher is charming and apparently open, and very easy to talk to, but he does not talk about deeper issues and feelings. His family does not think he can – and he does not regard it as the proper macho thing to do. This includes his epilepsy, which he rarely talks about.

'Jordan hates having epilepsy,' reports his mother, Anna. 'He went through a stage of being very frightened about it. I had to answer lots of questions about death. Can you die with your eyes open? What if you're still alive when they put you in the ground? Do people ever die in a seizure? He's just getting over that, but he still goes very withdrawn and remote. It's taking a lot of time for him to come to terms with having epilepsy.'

Twelve-year-old Michael describes his condition thus: 'I see my epilepsy as part of myself, like part of my hair colour. It's there – but there's no need to make a big fuss about it. I'm used to it.'

The normal hopes and fears of parents for their children may be poignantly accentuated for those with epilepsy in the family. Some families find that much of their life revolves around the child with epilepsy, and the condition influences their thoughts, fears and lifestyle, including outings and holidays. Many other parents feel strongly that epilepsy should not be allowed to rule their or their child's life, or be the key point in their identity.

Whatever you feel – and it is understandable that epilepsy will rule your life to some extent – these early years of a person's life are vital for forming her attitudes towards epilepsy, attitudes which play a vital part in overall self-esteem. Parents have a great deal of power when it comes to boosting confidence, and in encouraging the child to have a rich and varied self-image, not one which just focuses on epilepsy.

BABIES AND TODDLERS: FROM BIRTH TO FIVE

Case Study

Three-year-old Matthew was, frankly, unmanageable. He had tantrums if he did not get his own way, and getting him to go to bed took almost two hours every night. His parents, Tim and Melissa, were reluctant to discipline him because of his general poor health – he suffered frequent coughs, colds and infections, looked unwell all the time and had seizures when his temperature was at all raised. They were all too familiar with the desperate rush to the local hospital, and felt that the whole situation put an unacceptable burden on a small child. They accordingly overcompensated for his seizures, without realizing that this was already imposing on Matthew the psychosocial burden of being spoiled.

It is in these early years that children may be most at risk of what has been called 'the secondary gain of being ill', when the natural and overwhelming urge to protect a baby or toddler may spill over into anxious coddling, without parents even realizing it. One definition of being spoiled, by the renowned American paediatrician Berry T Brazelton, Emeritus Professor of Paediatrics at Harvard Medical School, is of an anxious, whiny child, searching for limits. According to Professor Brazelton, disciplining a child comes second only to love as a parental duty. Attending to your child's needs will not make her spoiled, but hovering over her, attending to her with anxiety, can end up creating insecurity and demanding behaviour – what we call being spoiled.

Professor Brazelton is talking about children in general; however, setting limits right from the start may be even more important for children with epilepsy because of the uncertainty and lack of control implicit in their condition. Depending on their temperament, they may need clear parental firmness even more than children in general. Discipline is a matter of providing limits and security, not punishing.

Save discipline for important matters, such as hot stoves. Keeping 'no' to a minimum and being consistent help a young child take discipline more seriously. Also fit the discipline to your child's age and stage of development. For example, do not worry about spoiling a baby under a year old. Generally, the younger a child, the more easily she will respond to being distracted – up to around three, she will not be able to reason well, or understand cause and effect clearly, so she may not understand the link between her behaviour and your reaction.

And do not wait for your child to misbehave. Gently try to teach her the sort of behaviour you expect in advance – for example, that you expect her to sit down for meals. Again, this varies according to age and development – do not expect too much! You should also reward good behaviour with attention, hugs and kisses.

Managing treatment

Case Study

Seven-year-old Nick was particularly averse to taking his medicine, as his mother, Maria, reported. 'I've tried everything – cutting chocolates in half and putting tablets in them, cutting the bottoms of yoghurt pots off and hiding tablets in them – you name it. Nick is developmentally delayed as well as having epilepsy, but for all his problems he's incredibly sharp and can tell at a glance when something's been tampered with. At one point I had to give him 26 different pills a day – it took over my whole life.'

Although Maria's difficulties, as described in the case study, are exceptional, they do point up the trials of having to give a small child medication. Many parents dislike this routine anyway, as it is a daily reminder that their child has epilepsy and has to take drugs. Also, drugs are often given in a sugary solution, and some parents worry about the effect of this on the teeth, although brushing well afterwards with a small dab of toothpaste is a good habit to get into and should prevent major problems. (As with any child, these early years are also a good time to start regular dental check-ups, but especially if your child takes medicine which contains sugar, or phenytoin, which can cause gum overgrowth as a side-effect.)

It is important that your child takes her medication, in order to prevent uncontrolled seizures, and parents may just have to display more willpower than their child. Ploys like mixing drugs with food or drink do work with some children. The other approach is simply to be tough and persistent – to keep on giving the medicine to the child until she gives in and accepts it as a set part of her daily routine – no matter how much she spits it out or cries meanwhile. This can be an upsetting and frustrating time for parents, but unfortunately you may have to show that it is one where there can be no bargaining.

■ Childproofing your home

Once babies become mobile, most parents are faced with the task of reorganizing their home, so early childhood is a good time to consider basic safety arrangements around the house. Many of the following suggestions apply whether your child has epilepsy or not, but some are specific to epilepsy.

- use safety plugs
- fit stair gates
- apply padding to sharp corners such as kitchen cupboards
- use cooker, radiator and fire guards
- fit smoke alarms
- fit safety locks on windows
- rehang toilet and bathroom doors so that they open outwards and will not be blocked if a child falls behind them
- ensure that shower cubicles are fitted with safety glass or plastic
- have windows and doors fitted with safety glass
- ensure that all medicines, including anti-epileptic drugs, are kept out of reach

There are many more ways in which to make your home safe. If you are concerned, contact an epilepsy support group for suggestions, or an accident prevention group such as the Royal Society for the Prevention of Accidents (*see* 'Useful Addresses').

Should your child have routine immunization?
Michael was fine up to 15–18 months, according to his mother, Jules. 'His problems started after he had his MMR [measles, mumps and rubella] jab – he stopped sleeping, his speech went backwards and he started having seizures. I don't know if there's any link – the doctors have always said it was probably coincidence and that it was going to happen anyway, but I've always thought about it and wondered.'

Whether to have a child immunized or not is a cause of great concern to many parents. Conventional medical opinion is that your child can have all the usual vaccinations safely, unless she has previously had an adverse reaction to a vaccination, or she is unwell at the time.

Some children do have febrile convulsions a week to ten days after the MMR vaccination, but this tends to be a 'one-off'. A few children may also have more seizures shortly after a vaccination, and perhaps a raised temperature and slight fever after the MMR.

The pertussis (whooping cough) vaccination is the one that tends to worry parents most because of its well-publicized association with brain damage. Medical research shows that the danger of brain damage and death is far greater from whooping cough than from the immunization, and that the more children are not immunized, the more likely this deadly disease is to return. In the UK, guidelines from the Department of Health, *Immunisation against Infectious Disease*, state that where there is a personal or family history of febrile convulsions, immunization is recommended, and doctors at the same time should give advice on preventing fever. Likewise, if there is a family history of epilepsy, immunization is still generally recommended. The American Academy of Pediatrics also strongly recommends that children receive their full set of immunizations. If you are concerned about your child having routine immunizations, consult your doctor.

Establishing good sleep patterns

It is worth trying to establish good sleep patterns from the start, given the fact that lack of sleep can be a seizure trigger. You might feel anxious or guilty about this, but undisturbed nights are vital for the whole family's wellbeing. You will manage much better if you are not exhausted and irritable from lack of sleep, and the chances are that your child will be sunnier-tempered and have more energy if she sleeps well too.

It may take time to get the message through to your child that night time is for sleeping, especially if she has multiple difficulties, but patience and consistency help. Set up a clear routine, with bedtime at about the same time, as it provides recognizable signals that the end of the day is approaching. Try to have a relaxed hour or so before bedtime so your child has a chance to wind down. A bedtime routine might include a bath, supper and a book in bed; massage (*see* page 114) also helps to relax some children before sleep.

With a baby or toddler who refuses to settle alone, you need to teach her new habits. One way of doing this is for you to settle her and sit by the bed, and then gradually withdraw from the room over a series of nights until she learns to settle alone. Night wakings also need consistent, firm handling, using the same settling methods as at bedtime, and keeping attention to a minimum so that your child is not rewarded for waking up.

A more rigorous approach, which is often recommended in sleep-training programmes, is the 'controlled crying' technique – saying goodnight to your child, leaving her to cry, and then coming back at frequent intervals to check her until she falls asleep. This could be something to discuss with your doctor if you feel it is appropriate for your child; you could also ask your doctor about any local sleep clinics, which are available in some areas specifically to help parents whose children have sleep problems.

Sometimes sleep may be complicated for your child by specific issues.

- Anxiety about her condition may appear as a common phobia (fear of the dark, monsters, burglars or witches, although it is normal for young children to have these fears anyway), or as specific fears (eg that she could die in her sleep from a seizure). These need to be discussed openly and sympathetically, and reassurance given.
- Some medications such as phenobarbitone can complicate sleep disturbances. Discuss this with your doctor; the timing or dosage may be changed, for example.
- Underlying brain dysfunction or damage may make sleep training slower but in the long run it will still be to your child's

benefit (and to yours). You may need specialized support from your doctor or a sleep training clinic, however.

• Sleeping medications often cause more sleep disturbances than they cure, as there can be a 'paradoxical response' to the medication which hypes your child up and leaves her less able to sleep. And medicines do not cure any night-waking habits she may have got into, or teach her to settle alone. Sleep experts generally stress that you should try behavioural approaches first. Sleep medication may be something to discuss with your doctor, perhaps as a temporary measure or as a back-up to sleep training; and it may be needed if your child has more severe developmental difficulties.

Massaging babies and toddlers
Touch is the most developed of the senses from birth, and massage, which is believed to stimulate the peripheral and autonomic nervous systems, has been shown to help a baby's breathing, boost the immune system and help digestion, as well as being very soothing. The association of health with massage goes back to Hippocrates, who believed that it was essential for doctors to be qualified in 'rubbing'. It is done from birth in many cultures throughout the world, such as some native American tribes, who massage their babies to stimulate their survival mechanisms and resist disease.

You do not need any special skills or equipment, just a warm room and a comfortable place for your child to lie. You can use baby oil, or basic oils such as grapeseed, sweet almond or coconut oil (do a 'patch test' on a small area of your child's skin first to make sure she does not suffer an allergic reaction) or essential oils such as lavender, Roman camomile or rose. Massage the main areas (abdomen, chest and back) from top to bottom and in a clockwise directions, and the arms and legs from top to bottom, with warm, well-oiled hands.

Do not massage your child if she is asleep, fretful or unwell, or if she has a skin problem or has had an immunization within the last couple of weeks. Consult your doctor if you are in doubt about massage for your child.

Childcare

If your child's epilepsy is straightforward and controlled, a competent childminder or babysitter should be able to manage without problems, although it is important that she is confident and happy about dealing with your child. You will need to explain your child's condition to her, along with any particular details concerning her care, what to do in the event of a seizure, and general management, as with any other child – snacks, naps etc.

Like other children your child will probably enjoy the stimulus and social benefit of going out to some form of daycare, such as mother and toddler group, playgroup or nursery. Again, so long as you talk her condition through thoroughly with carers, there should be no problems.

If your child has other difficulties in addition to her epilepsy, arranging daycare and babysitting will of course be more difficult, although no less essential. Many parents find themselves depending on their own families for support and time off. Otherwise, you could try to find out what outside help is available – in many places there are daycare nurseries for children with special needs.

SCHOOL YEARS: FROM 5 TO 12

This is the age when issues about overprotection and independence achieve a sharper edge as your child moves away from home and starts a new life at school. These years provide opportunities for encouraging independence in general areas as well as in epilepsy management, such as getting your child to take increasing responsibility for her medication – a particular area where good habits now can prevent problems later. At the age of 11, Barbara was developmentally delayed, but knew when she had not had her medication and would remind her parents of it when they were putting her to bed if they had forgotten the evening dose.

At this stage, it can be quite hard to start letting your child go. Up until school age it is quite natural for her to accompany you everywhere unless she is at nursery. But with school, a new life begins, which sooner or later sees the start of new needs and desires: to go round to a friend's house, to play in the street or to go on school trips. All sorts of questions arise during these years. When can your child walk to school alone? Should she be allowed to go to the shops by herself? When can she be left alone in the house for half an hour while you go out? Some doctors advise parents of children with well-controlled epilepsy to think and act as if the child were not going to have a seizure. They then just have to face the general concerns of all parents during these years, as the child gradually branches out into more freedom. How much independence your child should have does vary depending on her maturity and capability, and this can change quite quickly during this time – the seven-year-old you would not trust to go safely up the road to a neighbour's may be able to run to the corner shop on her own at eight.

Identity cards and bracelets, and epilepsy alarms, may make a difference to your child's confidence – and yours. For more information on where to get these, contact an epilepsy support association, or see under 'Useful Addresses'.

Case Study
Michael, aged 12, has an epilepsy alarm which, were he to fall in the street, would go off and say, 'I have epilepsy, please help me.' His mother, Jules, says, 'I can't tell you the difference this has made to our peace of mind. I still don't like him going out in the street to play on his bike with his friends, but having the alarm has made a great difference.'

School: educating the educators

Case Study
Michael's primary school had hardly even heard of epilepsy but became very keen to help in any way once they understood

what it was. 'I went in to help with reading,' recalls his mother, 'and I also met with the head and other teachers to explain what epilepsy was, and gave talks to the school. By the time he left they knew a lot about epilepsy – but now I find I'm having to start all over again with his junior school! They're slowly getting the idea. I work in the kitchens there as a cook, and I find it's often a question of saying no. No, he can't come home just because he doesn't feel well. No, I'm not taking him just because he says he's got a headache. No, he isn't allowed to get out of sports today. And, sometimes, no, he can't come home because he's had a seizure – he can have a rest and go back into class. I expect they think I'm very hard but I've learned through bitter experience that being tough and being consistent is the only way it works.'

Good communication between home and school is vital, and generally, the better informed a school is about epilepsy, the more supportive staff and pupils are likely to be. But while some schools have a clear policy on epilepsy, the condition may be totally new to others. While around 80 per cent of children with epilepsy attend ordinary schools and should be able to take part in most activities, lack of understanding at school can still be a problem and you may find that you have to 'educate the educators'. According to the British Epilepsy Association, two-thirds of children keep their condition secret from their school, one in three experiences difficulties in school from other children, and almost a quarter have some problems with teachers.

Make an appointment to see the head teacher, head of year, pastoral counsellor and/or class teacher. Some explanatory leaflets from a self-help organization might be useful – some groups produce material written specifically for teachers. The school might also welcome a talk on epilepsy from you, a member of a national organization or a specialist epilepsy nurse. It is important that your child's epilepsy is known to everyone with whom she has contact, including supervisory staff at breaks and mealtimes, volunteer helpers and office staff. Points to cover could be:

- the nature of your child's seizures – any aura or warning, exactly what happens and how long the seizure lasts, and (if you can) roughly how often they happen and whether they have any particular pattern or are triggered by anything in particular
- what to do about medication (the school may have a policy on this, though many modern anti-convulsants only need to be taken twice a day and so need not be taken into school)
- what to do in the event of a seizure, which means following the general guidelines as outlined in chapter 2, and the sort of attitude to take – if a teacher remains unflustered and supportive, the other children will accept the event much more easily
- what to do if there seems to be an emergency such as a prolonged seizure
- what to do after a seizure, such as letting your child rest for a set period of time – this should be clearly established to avoid future confusion, eg the school trying to send the child home every time she has a seizure
- any odd behaviour or daydreaming which should be noted by teachers
- whether the school needs more information on epilepsy
- how to handle peer reactions, and whether pupils would benefit from more details, say as part of a health education course

Your child herself may also have specific wishes, which should be respected. Teachers can have a massive influence on how children react, and an open, calm, positive attitude is essential.

You may well find that there are grey areas. What should staff do if your child complains of feeling unwell, or if they suspect her of using her epilepsy to get out of certain lessons? What about safety, for example in the sports field or in the science laboratory? Can the child attend swimming lessons? Is extra supervision available? Would it be appropriate for the parent to come in and help provide this supervision? Risk, success and failure are all needed for all children to learn and develop, but extra help may be needed from time to time. It can be a delicate balance to get right. The problems will vary according to the individual concerned, and it may take a period of trial and error to work out the best policy.

Teasing and bullying

Case Study

'At one point Mark had to wear a helmet because he was having a lot of drop attacks,' recalls his mother, 'so his school organized a hard hat day. Every child had to wear a hard hat for the day, and the school got everyone in – fire brigade, police, builders – everyone who had to wear a hat for work. It was brilliant. Mark's head teacher organized it all – he was wonderful.'

Some schools really rise to the occasion with a pupil who has epilepsy, and a thinking head teacher can inspire hundreds of children to real understanding and compassion. Unfortunately, however, children who appear a little different or vulnerable are more liable to bullying at school, and a label of epilepsy may be enough to provoke this. Some bullied children prefer to say nothing about it at home, but signs of the problem may be misbehaviour, temper tantrums or school refusal.

Find out what the school's policy on bullying is, and talk to your child's teacher and the head if necessary. You could offer to come in and give a talk on epilepsy and its realities, or arrange a speaker from a national self-help organization. It may also help to teach your child assertion techniques. The old differential between assertion and aggression holds good but it might do your child's confidence no harm if she is known to be a promising judo expert! More fundamental is inner confidence, which was discussed in chapter 2. By giving your child information on self-esteem, stress management and relaxation techniques, you may be giving her tools of real value when it comes to standing up to bullying and coming to terms with stressful relationships with peers.

Epilepsy and learning

Most children with epilepsy are as capable of learning as other children, but research does suggest that some do not perform up to ability. This could be for a variety of reasons and may sometimes need a formal assessment from an educational psychologist, health professionals and others. However, underachievement may have nothing to do with epilepsy, and could be something as simple as a poor general level of teaching. More specifically, it could involve:

- mistakenly low expectations of your child by teachers – and perhaps you
- teasing and bullying
- unrecognized absence seizures
- especially in more severe epilepsy, the side-effects of drugs or abnormal sub-clinical electrical activity in the brain which is not enough to produce a seizure but which does affect concentration and behaviour
- brain damage, however minimal, affecting just one area, such as reading
- poor memory – a common problem in children with epilepsy
- poor school attendance because of frequent seizures, especially if the school always sends the child home, or if parents keep the child off an extra day or two afterwards
- poor self-image and the fear of having seizures in front of others
- common problems such as home difficulties (divorce, bereavement) or difficulties with relationships with other children

Learning disabilities

Case Study
Joannie fell drastically behind with her reading at junior school, and the teachers expressed concern to her parents that she would not be able to go on to the secondary school of their choice. Her parents took her to a specialist, who quckly found that she had a very simple problem – she could not recognize phonics. In a few sessions this was overcome, her reading forged ahead and she caught up with the rest of her class.

Children with learning disabilities have a high incidence of epilepsy. Around 30 per cent of children with a learning disability have epilepsy; and, in those with a severe learning disability, this increases to 80 per cent. Most learning difficulties are mild and can be overcome quite quickly. A child is most likely to have serious learning difficulty if she has severe, uncontrolled seizures and/or physical and mental problems as well as epilepsy ('epilepsy plus').

If your child is falling seriously behind her peers, or if you think she is not getting all the help she needs at school, she may have special educational needs. You can contact your school to get a clearer picture of your child's individual requirements. Most children with special educational needs can attend an ordinary school, perhaps with the help of outside specialists, but sometimes a child with severe difficulties may do better at a special school, which can make specific provision for her needs. There are also a few schools just for children with epilepsy.

Social life

Outings and parties may require a little thought and planning, in which your child should be included.

- You have to decide together whether to tell the hosts about her epilepsy if they do not know. This may have added relevance if she has to take a dose of medicine in the evening.

- You should plan extra rest for your child beforehand if need be – parties can be exciting, and if she is sleeping over, the chances are that she and her friend will stay awake talking half the night.
- You might want to consider staying to help with a party if you are not totally confident about leaving your child.

However you manage it, it is very important that you encourage your child to have a good social life. Interaction with others is vastly confidence-boosting, and helps children learn to behave naturally with their peers, to gain social ease to see them through to adulthood and to forget about feelings of being 'different' which can be so isolating – indeed, disabling. Making friends, paying visits, being a hostess – all form a vital part of childhood, to the point where they could almost be said to form part of children's rights.

■ ADOLESCENCE: FROM 13 TO 18

The notorious problems of swinging emotions, self-doubt and rebellion are compounded by epilepsy for many teenagers. Epilepsy is the single most common neurological problem in adolesence, and in one American teenage clinic accounted for 60 per cent of all neurological problems.

While many teenagers have to cope with persisting epilepsy which started in childhood, this is also an age when it may be diagnosed for the first time, as in the case of JME, which often starts at around the age of 14 or 15. The type and frequency of seizures may also change because of the natural development of the type of epilepsy involved, or with the start of puberty and menstruation – for example, photosensitivity tends to peak in adolescence at about 16. The causes of epilepsy may also vary slightly in teenagers – for example, brain tumour, though rare, is more common than in younger children, and epilepsy is also more likely to result from head injury and abuse of drugs or alcohol. Less regular eating and sleeping habits, and an unwillingness to take prescribed drugs, can also affect the way your teenager's epilepsy progresses.

Should treatment be continued?

Around a third of all epilepsy which begins in childhood disappears of its own accord by puberty. So teenagers are often faced with the question of whether they should try and withdraw from their drug regimes and, if so, when. Drug taking itself often changes at this age. Apart from monitoring drug doses, which may need changing as the child grows, there is also the issue of compliance (*see* below).

This is often an uncomfortable time for teenagers as regards treatment. They may have to continue attending a paediatric clinic until a certain age (16 in the UK), where they may feel that their emotional and social concerns are not really covered; alternatively, they may dread leaving the familiarity of the clinic they have been attending for years, to move on to a neurologist for adults, who may not have a specialist interest in epilepsy.

Whether your child continues with her treatment or not depends on the type of epilepsy involved, and on the degree of seizure control. Generally, there is no way of predicting whether seizures will return or not, although some types of epilepsy, such as JME, are known to have a high rate of relapse (60–70 per cent) if drugs are withdrawn, while other types, such as BREC, naturally finish during these years. Although many doctors are optimistic about the 'safety blanket' of restarting drugs if need be, they may also feel obliged to warn teenagers that, rarely, seizure control may be more difficult to regain after a period in which drugs have been withdrawn.

Other factors need to be considered, such as whether exams or holidays abroad are pending – drug withdrawal usually takes at least two months, sometimes longer. Your child also needs to understand that a single seizure may result in her application for a driving licence being blocked (or an existing licence being lost), which may in turn threaten her job prospects.

Why teenagers may not take their anti-epileptic drugs
Non-compliance (not taking drugs as prescribed) is the most common cause of poor or lost seizure control – including status epilepticus – in teenagers, who may use this method to rebel against their condition and assert their independence. Although drugs give more independence, they are often seen as symbolic of dependence – some teenagers report feeling like 'junkies', others may feel that having to take medication makes them different from their peers, or may resent this artificial gateway to, or imposition of, 'normality'. Manipulating drug intake is also a way of asserting some control over a condition that feels completely beyond control.

Many teenagers also refuse to put up with side-effects – for example, teenage girls often stop taking sodium valproate because of hair loss and weight gain. Again, some teenagers will take less medication (or an extra dose) so that they can drink, which unfortunately only makes a seizure more likely. Some may feel the drugs do not work if they suddenly start having seizures again, or they may dislike feeling sleepy as a side-effect; both these reactions can happen as body size changes and dosage is adjusted.

Now is often a good time for a complete evaluation of diagnosis and treatment, including making sure your child understands the importance of medication – research shows that the better informed a child is, the more compliant she is likely to be.

If non-compliance is a problem with your child, try the following approaches.

- Suggest that she diverts her rebellious energy into exploring natural remedies such as healthy diet (with the usual provisos if possible of keeping up drug intake and not trying out any remedies prescribed by a natural therapist – eg herbs – without checking with her usual doctor).
- If a changed dosage is a problem, make sure she realizes that

the drugs can always be adjusted again until the right dosage level is found, so she should not hesitate to go back to the doctor.

- If side-effects are causing distress, your child's doctor may be able to switch to another drug.
- The prospect of entering a desired career or achieving a goal such as travel may also motivate some teenagers to take their medication.

Emotions

Case Study
Stuart, aged 17, was convinced his epilepsy was to blame for the fact that he did not have a girlfriend. One of his 'friends' had thrown out a chance comment to the effect that men with epilepsy were not able to have a sex life. A little education from his father and the family doctor set his mind at rest.

Emotional and sexual education, which are important for any teenager, take on added relevance for someone with epilepsy, who may need to be told quite clearly that her condition need not get in the way of relationships. In fact, although your child may not like to hear it, epilepsy can be a path to empathy in that it may make those affected more sensitive to others' feelings, more aware of their sufferings and so excellent candidates for being supportive friends.

Research suggests that teenagers with epilepsy may suffer low self-esteem, anxiety and depression – but so do those without epilepsy. The fact is that the condition often provides a peg on which to hang negative feelings of being unloveable and other problems and emotional hurdles. Some teenagers will need formal psychological support – do not ignore or show that you disapprove of persistent unhappiness. Many teenagers, whether they have epilepsy or not, go through a miserable phase at this time of life, and a little extra help from a professional counsellor could make a big long-term difference to their self-esteem, educational performance and general happiness.

On the positive side, coping with epilepsy may give your teenager more inner strength, and more ability to think for herself and withstand peer pressure. In particular, being confident and open about the condition seems to help – it is known that those who are able to talk about their epilepsy positively and appropriately are more successful at relationships. Do not forget that now more than ever your child will benefit from relaxation techniques and anything which helps combat stress and boost self-esteem.

▨ Teenage girls and epilepsy

A teenage girl may need specific advice as regards periods, contraception and family planning, because these can all be affected by epilepsy. It may seem early to start pre-conception counselling, but family planning is part of all teenagers' education, and there may occasionally be specific genetic issues which your child will have to consider. Also, some teenagers still believe (or may be told by others) that having epilepsy means that they will not be able to have children – so being open about such matters assumes even more importance.

Many teenage girls find they have more seizures around ovulation (which usually takes place roughly halfway through a cycle), or that their seizures cluster around menstruation (catamenial epilepsy). It is thought that this may be due to changes in the hormones oestrogen and progesterone, or to alterations in body fluids. Your doctor may prescribe extra medication in the week before menstruation, maybe in the form of an 'add-on' anti-epileptic such as clobazam, although this may cause drowsiness. Other options include the contraceptive pill to try to balance your daughter's hormones more, diuretics to reduce water retention, and increasing the usual dose of anti-epileptics just before a period. Some centres, especially in the USA, have tried treating catamenial epilepsy, as well as pre-menstrual syndrome (PMS), with natural progesterone and other hormonal therapies. Some people have also found that mood swings and seizures around periods can be improved by lifestyle changes – in particular, you might like to consider the advice on healthy eating and blood sugar swings in chapter 2. But be warned: if your daughter is considering alternative remedies for PMS, the often-recommended evening primrose oil has been reported by some as causing seizures, especially in those with temporal lobe epilepsy.

Girls need to be aware that some medication – carbamazepine, phenytoin and phenobarbitone – interact with the contraceptive pill, making it less reliable. Any bleeding between periods should be reported to your doctor as a sign that the contraceptive is probably not working.

It is important to make your daughter aware that, depending on the type of epilepsy she has, there may be a small risk of her children inheriting it. A genetic counsellor, trained in the science of genes and in psychology, can help her assess the chances more precisely, although she will not be able to make guaranteed predictions. For example, seizure threshold is part of a person's genetic make up, and may be passed on to children, but this is very variable. Mostly, the risk of passing on epilepsy to a child is very small, and more relevant if there is a question of a genetically inherited condition which can cause epilepsy, such as tuberous sclerosis.

A genetic counsellor will need a family medical history which is as full as possible, so parents can help their teenagers by writing down details of any illnesses or conditions in their own families that they are aware of.

Pre-conception advice is also important. Your daughter should be aware of a number of issues before she becomes pregnant. First, because anti-epileptic drugs deplete the supply of folic acid, women should take a higher than normal supplement of folic acid (4mg or 5mg per day), starting *before* conception, to prevent neural tube defects such as spina bifida.

The risks of anti-epileptic drugs to an unborn baby are

relatively small, and usually considered to be smaller than the risks of having several major uncontrolled convulsions, which can cause damage to the baby. All the same, your daughter should know that drugs can result in abnormalities, the most common one being cleft lip or palate, which accounts for about a third of abnormalities. However, the overall incidence of birth abnormalities is only 4 per cent more than the general population (around 2 per cent for the general population, 6 per cent for babies born to mothers on one anti-epileptic drug), and so is still very small. Doctors may be able to withdraw or change drugs during pregnancy. Drug levels will probably also need monitoring, as pregnancy itself sometimes triggers changes in seizure patterns.

Social life and late nights

The occasional late night is unlikely to do any harm, and your teenager needs to work out her own needs as regards sleep. Most people like to catch up on sleep after a late night, and it may also be possible for your child to plan other strategies to minimize the risks of loss of sleep. She should:

- try to get some extra sleep during the day before
- plan a quiet day or two afterwards
- go to bed half an hour earlier for a few days beforehand
- not worry – getting stressed or obsessional about how much sleep you have creates a whole new problem, and is counter-productive in terms of seizure control anyway

Your teenager certainly should not be frightened off socializing by a fear of any adverse effects, as a good social life remains as important now as ever.

Drinking

At some point your teenager will probably want to have a drink or two with her friends, and, as with all teenagers, this can be a good time to set up an attitude to alcohol which will carry her through into adulthood. So long as she continues to take her medication, eats sensibly and does not indulge in too many late nights, the odd social drink is unlikely to do her any harm, although she should check with her doctor if she is not sure how alcohol will interact with her medication.

Alcohol depresses the central nervous system and can lower the seizure threshold. It can also reduce the effect of anti-epileptic medication, so making a seizure more likely. Your child therefore needs to find her own tolerance level, but research suggests that drinking more than two units of alcohol in less than 12–15 hours significantly increases the risk of seizures in people. (A unit of alcohol is half a pint of beer or cider, a glass of wine or one measure of spirits such as whisky or gin.) Many seizures take place after drinking, sometimes as part of a hangover.

Large amounts of beer and cider are probably best avoided, as there is some evidence that too much fluid can cause seizures in some cases. Water intoxication has been mentioned as a particular feature of taking carbamazepine – people taking it may find their bodies may not be able to dispose of large quantities of fluid.

Epilepsy and alcohol
An American study of the link between alcohol and seizures found that the increased risk of having a first seizure begins at around four units of alcohol a day, with a risk factor of 1.2. The risk shoots to 3.0 for people drinking six to seven units a day, while people medically classed as alcoholics were 6.8 times more likely to have a first seizure than others.

Further education and careers

You and your teenager should consider further education and careers on just the same basis as everyone else – what would she like to do, what would she be good at and what qualifications does she have? But it may be advisable to give some thought to the matter at an earlier stage that normal, as a history of epilepsy can be a bar to some jobs, such as the armed forces or driving public transport vehicles. Careers such as nursing, teaching and childcare may also prove difficult if there is a recent history of seizures. Unfair though many of these restrictions are, and often due to outdated views of epilepsy, education and career concerns give yet another reason for your child to understand her epilepsy clearly, and to cultivate a positive outlook on it.

Independence and the future

There are many facets to independence at this age. A major one is driving. Regulations vary from country to country; in the UK, a person with epilepsy may drive if she has been seizure-free for a year, or has only had seizures in her sleep for the past three years. It may be galling for your teenager if she cannot drive, but on the other hand, with the increased enforcement of drink-drive laws, many people prefer to take taxis when going out for the evening anyway. Another advantage of not driving may be added fitness. All this may be little consolation when we live in a car culture, because your teenager is not *choosing* not to drive – it is being forced upon her by her health. However, perhaps in the long run she will be seen to be ahead of her times. Many people believe that the day of the car will have to pass for environmental reasons, and traffic accidents now represent the leading cause of death in children under 14 in the USA.

What is really at issue is your child's acceptance of her epilepsy as much as the driving itself. This means having responsibility for her own treatment, arranging regular check-ups and carrying a spare supply of medication. She could also join a national epilepsy support group, although obviously this kind of 'belonging' is not for everyone. Some people naturally prefer to establish relationships and get on with their lives in the privacy and anonymity most others take for granted, rather than getting together with other people just because of the joint bond of epilepsy.

Epilepsy organizations do have a powerful part to play in the future of epilepsy and its treatment, however. They are gradually forming what has been described as a 'subculture' of support which helps take individuals out of the isolation that the condition all too often brings. This may reflect an organic and growing feeling that it is time for people with epilepsy to band together and acquire a recognizable status and definable rights, and that this type of 'people power', as well as providing much-needed companionship, is the best way to change any remaining outdated public attitudes, or even laws.

Conclusion

Towards a better quality of life

With the increasing recognition that epilepsy management is more than seizure control, quality of life has been receiving more attention than ever before in the last few years. A recent US Department of Health national health interview survey looked at quality of life in more than 11,000 children aged 6–17. The overwhelming suggestion from the findings was that poor psycho-social adjustment in children with epilepsy is the result of self-fulfilling prophecies stemming from the way parents react to the condition. The researchers concluded that parents may unintentionally create or worsen poor psycho-social adjustment in their children by being overprotective, rejecting or having low expectations for them. Obviously, this places a huge onus on parents to examine their own attitudes to their children and epilepsy. However, on the positive side, it does suggest that a good quality of life can be achieved with the back-up of parents who know how and when to let their children go, while at the same time accepting and supporting them as they are, and encouraging them to aim high.

As well as parental attitudes being an influence, quality of life can also be affected by medical factors such as underlying brain dysfunction and anti-epileptic medication. In addition, it can be affected by others' perceptions of epilepsy, and the way epilepsy impacts on self-confidence and social life. In another American study, epilepsy researcher Joan Austin compared quality of life in children aged 8–12 with epilepsy with that of children with asthma. Overall quality of life in terms of psychological, social and school factors was found to be poorer in the children with epilepsy. Four years later, Austin and her colleagues again compared quality of life in the two groups. They found that overall quality of life was still poorer for the adolescents with epilepsy than for those with asthma. The study suggests that epilepsy still carries a relatively greater social stigma, which can adversely affect quality of life.

Attitudes have improved in recent years as the public learn more about epilepsy. All the same, families frequently remain weighed down by cultural baggage, in particular the fear of what others will think of their child's epilepsy. In fact, attitudes vary widely and, on the whole, the better informed people are, the more accepting and understanding they are likely to be. Fear of the unknown often lies behind public negativity – 'If someone says he has epilepsy, does that mean he's going to start thrashing about right now in front of me?' Others may fear the loss of control mainfested by a seizure, and may lack the mechanisms to deal with this involuntary suspension of the social self. These kinds of fears can often be allayed by parents being open about their child's epilepsy. Sharing medical information with schools, friends, neighbours and officials can be a positive way to deal with stigma.

In recent years, increasing awareness of epilepsy has led to society learning to accept and deal with epilepsy as a medical condition which can be treated. It is now also increasingly accepted that quality of life goes beyond treating the seizure disorder, and means paying attention to the child and his general quality of life. It may seem unfair that public ignorance about epilepsy should put the onus on parents to change matters, but it does give you good reason to inculcate a positive, self-reliant attitude in your child, rather than encouraging him, however subtly, to view himself as a victim of a disorder over which he has no control. The more open and positive you can be about epilepsy, the more the culture will change for the better, and the better the prospects will be for children with the condition in the future.

Further Reading

Appleton, Richard and Richard Gibbs, *Epilepsy in Childhood and Adolescence*, Martin Dunitz, London, 1995

Appleton, Dr Richard E, Brian Chappell and Margaret Beirne, *Your Child's Epilepsy – A Parent's Guide*, Class Publishing, London, 1997

Brazelton, Dr T Berry, *Your Child's Emotional and Behavioural Development*, Penguin, London, 1995

Brostoff, J and L Gamlin, *The Complete Guide to Food Allergy and Intolerance*, Bloomsbury, London, 1989

Carter, Jill and Alison Edwards, *The Elimination Diet Cookbook*, Element, Shaftesbury, 1997

Chadwick, D and S Usiskin, *Living with Epilepsy*, 2nd edition, Macdonald Optima, London, 1991

Fenwick, Dr P and Elizabeth, *Living with Epilepsy*, Bloomsbury, London, 1996

Ferber, Dr Richard, *Solve Your Child's Sleep Problems*, Dorling Kindersley, London, 1989

Freeman, John M, Eileen P G Vining and Diana J Pillas, *Seizures and Epilepsy in Childhood – A Guide for Parents*, Johns Hopkins University Press, Baltimore, 1997

Freeman, John M, Millicent T Kelly and Jennifer B Freeman, *The Epilepsy Diet Treatment – An Introduction to the Ketogenic Diet*, Demos Publications, New York, 1997

Goffman, Erving, *Stigma*, Prentice-Hall, Englewood Cliffs, NJ, 1963

Hanscomb, A and L Hughes, *Family Health Guide: Epilepsy*, Ward Lock, London, 1995

Holford, Patrick, *The Optimum Nutrition Bible*, Piatkus, London, 1997

Hopkins, Anthony and Richard Appleton, *Epilepsy – The Facts*, 2nd edition, Oxford University Press, Oxford, 1996

Laidlaw, Mary and John Laidlaw, *People with Epilepsy – How They Can Be Helped*, Churchill Livingstone, London, 1984

Lindenfield, Gael, *Confident Children*, Thorsons, London, 1994

Oxley, Jolyon and Jay Smith, *The Epilepsy Reference Book*, Faber & Faber, London, 1991

Rowlands, Barbara, *The Which? Guide to Complementary Medicine*, Which? Books, London, 1997

Sacks, Oliver, *Migraine*, Picador, London, 1993

Sander, L and P Thompson, *Epilepsy – A Practical Guide to Coping*, Crowood Press, Marlborough, Wilts, 1989

Scambler, Graham, *Epilepsy*, Tavistock/Routledge, London, 1989

Schneider, Joseph W and Peter Conrad, *Having Epilepsy – The Experience and Control of Illness*, Temple University Press, Philadelphia, 1983

Temkin, Owsei, *The Falling Sickness*, Johns Hopkins University Press, Baltimore, 1945

Thomas, Caroline, *Epilepsy – A Holistic Approach*, Images Publishing, 1993 (Available from Nutricentre, 7 Park Crescent, London W1N 3HE)

Too, Lilian, *Feng Shui, Health*, Element, Shaftesbury, 1998

Vickers, Andrew, *Complementary Medicine and Disability – Alternatives for People with Disabling Conditions*, Chapman & Hall, London, 1993

Walker, Dr M C and Professor S Shorvon, *Understanding Epilepsy*, Family Doctor Publications, in association with the British Medical Association, London, 1995

Walker, Peter, *Baby Massage*, Piatkus, London, 1995

Weller, Stella, *Yoga for Children*, Thorsons, London, 1996

Wildwood, Chrissie, *Flower Remedies*, Element, Shaftesbury, 1994

—— *The Complete Guide to Reducing Stress*, Piatkus, London, 1997

Xuan, Sheila and Ke Song, *Traditional Chinese Medicine*, Hamish Hamilton, London, 1995

The British Epilepsy Association provides leaflets and videos on several aspects of epilepsy. The National Society for Epilepsy also has a video and leaflet information package on epilepsy in general (*see* 'Useful Addresses').

Useful Addresses

International

International Bureau for Epilepsy
PO Box 21
NL-2100 AA Heemstede
Holland
Tel: 23 29 10 19, fax: 23 47 01 19
(An international organization for people with epilepsy and their friends)

International League against Epilepsy (ILAE)
Department of Health and Human Services
National Institute of Health
Building 31
Bethseda
Maryland 20892
USA
(For doctors and other professionals)

Europe

Associazione Italiana contra l'Epilepsia
Via Copernico 28
400 58 Malalbergo
Bologna
Italy
Tel: 336 595 463, fax: 10 555 6603

Bureau Français de l'Epilepsie
236 bis rue de Tolbiac
75013 Paris
France
Tel: 1 53 606 664, fax: 1 45 300 809

Danske Epilepsiforening
Dr Sellsvej 28
DK 4293 Dianalund
Denmark
Tel: 58 26 44 66, fax: 58 26 44 51

Deutsche Epilepsie Vereinigung
Zillestrasse 102
10585 Berlin
Germany
Tel: 30 342 4414, fax: 30 342 4466

Epilepsie Selbsthilfegruppen Osterreichs
Haupfstr. 44/2/2
2344 Ma. Enzersdorf
Austria

Epilepsie Vereniging Nederland
PO Box 270
3990 GB Houten
The Netherlands
Tel: 30 63 440 63, fax: 30 63 440 60

Epilepsyaliitto
Kalevankatu 61
00180 Helsinki 18
Finland
Tel: 0 694 8433, fax: 0 694 9927

Epilepsy Association of Iceland
Poysbox 5182
126 Reykjavik
Iceland
Tel: 1 5514570, fax: 1 5514580

Greek National Association Against Epilepsy
Aghia Sophia Children's Hospital
Dept. Of Neurology/Neurophysiology
Athens 11527
Greece
Tel: 1 7771 811, fax: 1 7705 785

Les Amis de la Ligue Nat. Belge contra l'Epilepsie
Avenue Albert 135
Brussels 1060
Belgium
Tel: 2 3443263

Liga Nacionale Portuguesa contra a Epilepsia
Rua Sa da Bandeira 162–1 o
4000 Porto
Portugal
Tel: 200 56 03, fax: 2 302 515

Schweizerische Liba gegen Epilepsie
c/o Pro Infirmis
Postfach 1332 8032 Zurich
Switzerland
Tel: 1 383 5455, fax: 1 383 3049

Spanish Epilepsy Association
Calle Escuelas Pias 89
Barcelona 08017
Spain
Tel: 3 3495400

Australia

National Epilepsy Association
P O Box 224
Parramatta
NSW 2150
Tel: 2 891 6118, fax: 2 891 6137

Canada

Epilepsy Canada
1470 Peel Street
Suite 745
Montreal
Quebec
H3A 1T1
Tel: 514 845 7855, fax: 514 845 7866

Montreal Neurological Institute
3801 University Street
Montreal
Quebec
H3A 2B4

New Zealand

New Zealand Epilepsy Association Inc
P O Box 1074
Hamilton
Tel: 7 834 3556, fax: 7 834 3553

South Africa

South African National Epilepsy League
P O Box 73
Observatory 7935
Tel: 21 473014, fax: 21 4485053.

United Kingdom

British Complementary Medicine Association
9 Soar Lane
Leicester
LE3 5DE
Tel: 0116 242 5406

British Epilepsy Association
Anstey House
40 Hanover Square
Leeds
LS3 1BE
Tel: 0113 243 9393, fax: 0113 242 8804, e-mail: epilepsy@bea.org.uk,
helpline: 0800 30 90 30

British Holistic Medical Association
Roland Thomas House
Royal Shrewsbury Hospital South
Shrewsbury
SY3 8XF
Tel: 01743 261155

Council for Complementary and Alternative Medicine
Park House
206–208 Latimer Road
London
W10 6RE
Tel: 0181 968 3862

Epilepsy and the Young Adult (EYA)
13 Crondace Road
London
SW6 4BB

Epilepsy Bereaved?
P O Box 1777
Bournemouth
BH5 1YR

For a Better Life with Epilepsy (FABLE)
The Old Bank
239–241 Crookes
Sheffield
S10 1TF
Tel: 0800 521 629 (helpline), tel/fax: 0114 268 4977

National Society for Epilepsy
Chalfont St Peter
Gerrards Cross
Bucks
SL9 0RJ
Tel: 01494 873991, fax: 01494 871927

Royal Society for the Prevention of Accidents (RoSPA)
Edgbaston Park
353 Bristol Road
Birmingham
B5 7ST
Tel: 0121 248 2000

USA

The Epilepsy Foundation of America
4351 Garden City Drive
Landover
Maryland 20785–4941
Local phone: (301) 459 3700, toll free: (800) EFA-1000, fax: (301) 577–2684

The Charlie Foundation
501 10th Street
Santa Monica
California 90402
(Information and support on the ketogenic diet)

Comprehensive Epilepsy Center
New York Hospital – Cornell Medical Center
525 East 68th Street
New York
NY 10021
Tel: (212) 746 2359
(Surgery specialists)

Pediatric Epilepsy Center
The Johns Hopkins Medical Institutions
Meyer 2-147
600 North Wolfe Street
Baltimore
Maryland 21287-7247

Rasmussen Syndrome Resource Group
8235 Lethbridge Road
Millersville
Maryland 21108
Tel: (410) 987 5221

Index

Note: where more than one reference is given, main references are indicated in **bold**

immune system 14–15, 53
immunization 20, **111–12**
independence 116, 130
infantile spasms *see* West syndrome
Institute for Optimum Nutrition
(ION) 53
involving your child 38
iron deficiency 85–6

Jacksonian seizures 8
Janz syndrome *see* Juvenile
myoclonic epilepsy
jerking movements 7, 9, 11
Juvenile myoclonic epilepsy (JME)
11, 22, 122, 123

Ketogenic diet 5, 12, 13, **79–84**
ketosis 80

Lamotrigine 66
Landau-Kleffner syndrome (LKS)
13, 23
learning and epilepsy 120
learning disability 24, 44–5, 121
Lennox-Gastaut syndrome 10,
12–13, 73
life force (qi) 97, 98, 99, 100, 102,
104
low self-esteem 125–6

magnesium deficiency 53, 84–5
Magnetic Resonance Imaging (MRI)
61–2
malabsorption syndrome 84, 88
manganese 53, 86
massage 48, 96–7, 100, 102, **114**
measles, mumps and rubella (MMR)
vaccination 20–1, 111–12
medical assistance 55
medical history 59
medication
and behavioural problems 44
and contraceptive pill 127
as seizure control 56–7
as seizure trigger 27
and under fives 110

see also drug treatments
meditation 49
meningitis 11, 12, 19
menstruation 126–7
migraines 16, 88
mineral deficiencies 53, 85–6
misdiagnosis 15–18, 23
monitoring treatment 64–5
mood swings 36, 53, 92, 127
MRI spectroscopy 72
multiple subpial transection (MST)
74
muscle jerks 7, 9, 11
music therapy 46, 50
myoclonic seizures 7, 11

naturopathy 94
neuronal migration disorders 21
neuropsychological tests 63, 72
neurotrophin-4 (NT-4) 22
non-compliance 124
non-convulsive seizures 7, 9, **54**
non-epileptic attacks (NEAs) 17
nutrition **51–3**, 84–6

occipital lobe of brain 9
operations 73–4
organizations 131
osteopathy 93, 94
outgrowing epilepsy 29–30
overprotection 31–2, 108–9

pallid syncopal attacks 15
parental attitudes 132
parents 47–51
parietal lobe of brain 9
partial (focal) seizures 6, **8**, 10–11,
73–4, 96
periods 26
pertussis (whooping cough) 112
'petit mal' 7–8
phenobarbitone 113
phenytoin 65, 66
photosensitive epilepsy 11, 27–8
physical exercise 49